Excerpts from Letters to the Author

"Just writing you a quick note to share the PHENOM-ENAL news: I am 7 months pregnant, due in May!!! We are having a baby boy and to quote you in your book, I'm having an "uneventful" pregnancy at 42 and we conceived ON OUR OWN!! After being told my AMH was too low and my FSH was too high. My love and gratitude for your support and love and for teaching me SO much about my body and my spirit. You were one of the ONLY people in my life that encouraged me and knew that something fabulous was possible for me, whether it came through a biological pregnancy or another way. Your voice on those calls and your book and your workshop kept me going when I felt like I had little else. And yes, I was encouraged as well, to go straight to egg donor, which I resisted, obviously. You gave me faith in my body when few others even considered a natural pregnancy to be possible.

I will never forget when you looked at me in your workshop in Woodstock and said, "Ronda, WHEN you're a mother... NOT IF!" Figured Valentine's Day was a great day to share the love. Thank you from the bottom of my heart."
— Ronda White, Rockwall, TX

"I have been wanting to write to you for some time now to share with you the news that I am pregnant! I want to thank you ever so much for your huge role in helping me arrive at this wonderfully exciting and miraculous stage! Your work is absolutely phenomenal! I feel extremely fortunate to have been able to attend your workshop; and your books and teleconferences provide much needed guidance, support & encouragement to the many women out there

who feel isolated and despondent."
 – Kate Strever, Greenwich, CT

"Just a short note to tell you that the unbelievable has happened: I got pregnant naturally. Your April 15th workshop happened to be in the fertile time of my cycle and the magic happened! I attribute this natural pregnancy to the journey I have started through your books and your work. Attending your workshop has confirmed my wish not to do a third IVF; has made me less doubtful and made me understand your tools really well. Discovering your work last October has literally changed and saved my life, and not only on the baby making level. I think your work goes much deeper than that. I didn't know you when I first read your books but I knew that there was somebody very intelligent, articulate and determined behind these writings and that really spoke to me. I will continue exploring my journey through your tools and once again, I would like to thank you for your wonderful work."
 – Julie-Anne Derome, Quebec, Canada

"Dear Julia, I came from Switzerland last summer to attend your workshop. After many fertility specialists telling me my only chance at motherhood would be through egg donation or adoption, I was compelled to come. I was diagnosed with early menopause, I had had three miscarriages along the way, and began blaming myself for having "old eggs" and "waiting too long." I was 38 at the time. The day with you was transformative. I was filled with such energy and passion...Three months later I became pregnant. I get goose bumps now even typing this. The doctors were completely stunned and kept doing ultrasounds every week in the beginning to "see if it was still there." They didn't believe it could possibly be viable, yet I went on to have a normal pregnancy and deliver a healthy baby boy on June 19. Keep up your wonderful work, Julia! You are an inspiration, and we can't thank you enough."

  – Amy Smearsoll, La Tour-de-Peilz, Switzerland

"Julia, your path of allowing the truth to unfold has been a blessing to me and now my family, My Fertile Heart work has been strong and ongoing through our adoption journey and our time together on the teleconference calls has continued to impact me greatly. Your courage in the world is so good and inspiring!"

  – Michele Jasmin Sanders, Santa Fe, New Mexico

"I have been meaning to write you to tell you that I became pregnant in January at age 43, after more than 2 1/2 years of trying to conceive and dealing with secondary infertility, blood clotting, and miscarriages. There is no doubt in my mind that your visualizations and other ideas and beliefs in your books and workshop helped me to conceive the gorgeous little boy I now have. I want to thank you from the bottom of my heart."

  – Lisa Pinard, Washington, D.C.

"I just wanted to send you a quick note of thank you for helping me hold onto hope and "turn right down the tree filled avenue leading to the park full of possibility" when I was quite often tempted to "turn left down the path of hopelessness and self pity." I am now 4 months pregnant and just starting to show after being told I was post menopausal at

the age of 34 by 3 different fertility specialists, with my last FSH reading over 150 and my anti mullerian under 0.01! Both your books and your teleconferences helped me to hold onto the empowered "fertility specialist within" and to keep going. I thank you from the bottom of my heart!"
— Kumari Linley, London, UK

"I am writing to share that I am pregnant! I am 32 weeks today! This baby is a miracle for us. I turned 44 in May and have experienced 3 miscarriages prior to this pregnancy. We went through 3 failed IVF cycles. This will be our first child. I wanted to thank you, Julia, for your books, the workshop and the teleconferences...I think that all of it had a cumulative effect in helping me create this baby. The workshop in particular really helped me to not give up and to believe that my "assignment" was to do the work and to believe that I could create a healthy baby. What you wrote in your books, talked about in the workshop and the teleconferences were like medicine for me."
— Louise Lawson, Boston, MA

"Our very perfect daughter, Annabelle Katherine Queally greeted the world this past Friday. As you know this was a long, long journey of exploratory surgery, failed IUI's and Clomid cycles. IVF would've been our next step before we found you. There are no words to fully describe our love for Annabelle, nor are there words to thank you for helping to guide us through the journey that brought her to us. It was a magical moment for me tonight, to be sitting breastfeeding our baby on the same couch where I spent so many hours listening to your voice on the Fertile Heart Imagery CD."
— Mandy Queally, Yarmouth, ME

"Four years ago, I read your book, took your workshop and followed up with two phone consults with you. I was transformed. After ten years of hormonal imbalance, right after your workshop my cycles started to become regular, and during the private sessions we've really hit on the crux of my long-standing anxiety. I diligently practiced with your Imagery CD and practiced Body Truth. And thanks to the effect of the workshop on my cycles I was able to begin IVF which was successful. I had twins nine months after your workshop and 22 months later had a surprise baby without the use of medical intervention. You helped me connect the deep yearning for a child with other original needs."
— Alisyn Camerota, New York, NY

"By the time I read your books I had six failed IVF's and a number of miscarriages. With every miscarriage my desperation was increasing to unbearable levels. Since the medical community offered me very few options I knew that I was going to have to make something change inside of me, but I had no idea how to do that. I've been in therapy for years and tried every alternative treatment but I was still stuck. The Fertile Heart tools, the workshops and your books opened a whole new way of thinking and feeling about this journey. They taught me how to gradually become my own Ultimate Mom. I don't think that our miracle baby would be here today without the Fertile Heart Ovum work and your support and love."
— Leslie Zarra, New York, NY

Professional Praise

"This remarkable book (The Fertile Female) gives inspiration and focus to couples trying to achieve their goals. Written by an experienced and sensitive caregiver it should be read by patients and their doctors."
 – Jonathan Scher, M.D., author Preventing Miscarriage: The Good News.

"It's nice to read a medical story with a happy ending. It's even nicer when we learn something useful from it for our own lives. So it is with Julia Indichova's mindful journey described in Inconceivable."
 – Ellen Langer, PhD, Professor of Psychology Harvard Medical School, author of Mindfulness.

"A most valuable resource not only for women but also for their partners. The Fertile Female is a thoughtful, passionate and loving guide to the intangibles that surely contribute to difficulty in conceiving."
 – Marc Goldstein M.D., F.A.C.S. Surgeon-in-Chief M.D. F.A.C.S. Male Reproductive Medicine and Surgery, Cornell Institute for Reproductive Medicine, author of The Couples Guide to Fertility.

Julia Indichova is the 'Rocky' of the fertility world. Her willingness to explore every possible alternative is remarkable. Her story is another brilliant example of the impact of the mind-body connection."
 – Richard Mars, M.D. Medical Director, Center for Assisted Reproductive Medicine, Santa Monica UCLA Medical Center, author of The Fertility Book.

"I would love all my patients to fight for themselves with the strength of Ms. Indichova's commitment. Her demanding self-analysis, good humor, and determination just fly off the page. It's magic."
– Alan Natow, M.D. clinical Associate Professor, New York University School of Medicine

"When inspiration and information are combined there is no limit to what one may create. Read this (Inconceivable) and learn that what you can conceive of can be achieved."
– Bernie Siegel, M.D., bestselling author of Love, Medicine and Miracles

"This revealing narrative (Inconceivable) shows that for some individuals a positive mind-set and alternative medicine may be as powerful as traditional fertility drugs."
– Sami David, M.D. Gynecologist/Fertility Specialist, co-author of Making Babies

the fertile female

How the Power of Longing

for a Child

Can Save Your Life

and

Change the World

Julia Indichova

Author's Note: To safeguard the anonymity of the women and
men whose stories appear in this book, names and identifying
details have been changed. The details of their work with the
Fertile Heart™ tools and the manner in which they healed,
conceived and brought their children home, has not been al-
tered.

*The ideas and tools offered are not meant to replace the
advice of an appropriate health professional; they are
shared with the understanding that each reader accepts
full responsibility for her/his well being.*

Library of Congress Catalog Card Number: 2006927765
ISBN-10: 0-9660078-7-5
ISBN-13: 978-0-9660078-7-9

Book design by Edward Baum

Manufactured in the United States of America

10 9 8 7 6 5 4 3

Excerpt from *Life Is a Miracle* by Wendell Berry, copyright@2000. Reprinted
by permission of Counterpoint, a member of Perseus Books, L.L.C

Only brief phrases which meet the "fair use" standard are quoted from other
works covered by copyright law.

Library of Congress Cataloging-in-Publication Data
Indichova, Julia The Fertile Female:How the Power of Longing for a Child
Can Save Your Life and Change the World – 1ˢᵗ ed.
1. Infertility – Female – Popular works.2.Infertility, Female –Psychological
aspects. 3.Conception – Nutritional Aspects. 4.Fertility, Human – Psychological aspects.

for my husband
mother father sister brother
friend
Edward Nathan Baum

and

for all the
women
and
men
who follow their longings
with
wide open
eyes

Contents

the fertile female

Introduction

As Fertile as It Gets

"The most radical influence of reductive science has been the virtually universal adoption of the idea that the world, its creatures, and all the parts of its creatures are machines – that is, that there is no difference between creature and artifice, birth and manufacture."

– *Wendell Berry, Life is a Miracle*

"…there are a hundred paths through the world that are easier than loving.
But, who wants easier?"

– *Mary Oliver, White Pine*

Last summer a tree in our backyard was struck by lightning. Only a stump remained standing; the rest of the massive trunk lay sprawled on the ground. Looking at it, you'd say: firewood. We're not the best of groundskeepers, and the following spring, the tree was still there. One Monday morning I noticed a tiny apple blossom on one branch. A few days later several more boughs glistened with white. A single thread of the trunk remained attached to the root, just enough for those blossoms to press through.

Our longing for a child is often our one remaining strand of connection with the part of us that insists on staying alive – the place where our passions are still intact. I am writing this book for anyone who feels such a longing and wishes to harness it; to see it as an invitation to roll up our sleeves and discover that change is possible, that what we feel and believe about ourselves and the world, and the action we choose to take, can make a difference.

Fifteen years ago, my yearning for a second child led me to follow an entirely unfamiliar trail, a path that revealed a landscape more stunning than anything I'd ever seen. Wildflowers, hidden waterfalls, berries ripe for picking at every turn. Awed by my discovery, I called to everyone within earshot: Come, you've got to see this!

This call to others was my first book, *Inconceivable*. It was meant to invite the reader on the pilgrimage I took

– with all its initial doubts, disappointments, and sudden insights – in the hope that they too would be changed by it. Judging from the letters I've received over the last several years, that is, amazingly, what happened.

A number of women and couples who read *Inconceivable* began to call for more guidance. A small Sunday afternoon support circle, and a series of seminars that later became the Fertile Heart Conceptions workshops, emerged in response. In this book I am attempting to document all I've learned in the last fifteen years, to share the many stories of the women I've worked with, and to hand you the tools that helped them decode the messages behind their symptoms.

For readers in their late thirties, forties, or older, may this book, above all, help you resist the temptation to blame yourself for the life choices you've made so far. May it strengthen your commitment to pursue motherhood without succumbing to the collective hysteria of the last good egg. The question of statistical probabilities is just not that interesting to me. In the last decade I've seen countless women give birth in spite of overwhelming odds; apparently none of these babies was up on the latest research on ovarian reserve, morphology, or fragmented embryos.

By no means do I wish to imply that the difficulties we come up against are to be taken lightly, or that scientific research is to be dismissed. But when it comes to pursuing motherhood, the questions that make a lot more sense than statistics are these: Am I willing to discover what this longing for a child is about for me? Can I let it become the invisible umbilical cord already attached to my heart? Am I able to trust that no matter what happens, following that longing can only enlarge my life?

For the younger reader, I hope this book becomes an ally in learning to distinguish between the reality of your biological clock and the self-hating mechanism, egged on by a myriad of societal influences, of turning that clock into a time bomb.

I can speak about this form of coercion from direct experience. As an aspiring actress I spent most of my twenties struggling to financially support myself. My elderly father, a recent immigrant, propelled by his own powerlessness and a wish to see me settled, never missed an opportunity to remark, "You know, once a woman hits thirty, something happens; somehow the flush of youth just isn't there anymore.

"Well," he'd add mournfully, sliding his reading glasses back over his eyes and returning to his crossword puzzle, "maybe having children is not all that important."

After one of these exchanges I would go home, stare at my reflection in the bathroom mirror, and count the growing number of fine lines under my eyes. Then I'd resolve to attend every singles event on this side of the Atlantic. My growing desperation made all able-bodied males run for cover.

The one thing my father didn't tell me was that unless I learned to love and take care of myself first, I was less than likely to end up in a happy union.

By a sheer act of grace, in the form of extensive therapy, a few good friends, and countless consciousness-raising adventures, I began to follow my own truth. My father's voice grew more faint, and a new voice emerged inside me – a voice I slowly came to recognize as my own.

I guess I might as well confess my bias right at the start: In the range of human experiences, motherhood, for me, is very near the top of the list. But motherhood will not save your life.

To let all that comes – the difficult and the easy – move through you, and to respond to it as truthfully as you can,

can not only save your *own* life, it can heal generations' worth of grief in your family line. And it can help you find the courage to speak up and add to the Power of Good.

To be aware of the role each of us plays in the ongoing creation of our own lives, our children's lives, and the world, and to participate with our eyes wide open, is about as fertile as any of us could ever hope to become.

Part One

Problems and Mysteries

Chapter One

The Zen of Baby Making

"Life is a mystery to be lived, not a problem to be solved"

– Soren Kirkegaard, *Fear and Trembling*

*I*n ancient China there lived a farmer, who was considered wealthy and blessed. He had land, a robust young son, and a horse to help him with his plowing,. One day the horse ran off. "What a curse!" exclaimed the villagers. But all the farmer said was, "Maybe." The next day the horse returned, leading an entire herd of wild mustangs. All the neighbors gathered around, celebrating the farmer's good fortune. "Maybe," he replied. The following morning the farmer's son tried to break in one of the wild horses; the mustang threw him and the young man broke his leg. "Without the help of your son, you can't plant your fields. What misfortune!" lamented the villagers. "Maybe," said the farmer. A week later the emperor's soldiers stormed into town, enlisting all the young men for war. The farmer's son couldn't go. His broken leg made him unfit for battle. When the rest of the village marveled at our farmer's extraordinary luck, the only thing he said was "Maybe."

– Chinese folktale

In the course of a lifetime, great teachers appear to each of us in a myriad of ways. Sometimes we come upon them at the peaks of the Himalayas, and sometimes they show up on our doorstep as a number on a lab report.

When I was first told that my soaring hormone levels had narrowed down my childbearing options to zero, the idea of a life-changing opportunity did not enter my mind. After years of pursuing neurosis as a primary career (the theater world provided an ideal setting for such efforts), I was finally married, had a beautiful, healthy child and liked my job. As far as I was concerned, the years of searching for answers were over.

When the diagnosis arrived, all I wanted was for someone to fix me as quickly as possible. My plan was to assemble a team of the best and the brightest, who would somehow track down and capture that last fertilizable egg before my next birthday, then attend to the mechanics of turning that egg into a baby. The only crimp in my plan was that none of my doctors seemed to want to go along with it.

The panic and despair that set in seemed selfish, and inappropriate. Why does it hurt so much, I thought, when I already have the most wonderful child in the world? Reading stories of childless couples in my various self-help books, I felt as though I was getting in line for seconds before everyone had been served. And yet each morning I'd wake up with an image of Ed, Ellena, and myself sitting around the dining room table waiting for someone; loving one another deeply but sad because someone was missing.

In those days my holistic approach to health consisted of finding an acupuncturist and ordering brown rice instead of white at the local Chinese restaurant. Endless bowls of brown rice and five acupuncturists later I found a homeopath, then a Native American medicine man, an herbalist, a midwife, and a number of wise women and men of all healing traditions. I had replaced the experts at fertility clinics with the experts in Chinatown and *environs*.

One day, as I was leafing through diet and juicing books

at the local health food store, a most surprising idea came. An epiphany. I realized *I* had an opinion about the diagnosis, plus a glimmer of a thought for a possible solution. The coming months brought the greatest growth spurt of my forty-three years. Carefully I reviewed all information given to me by my doctors and various healers, and did a great deal of research of my own, and one step at a time, a healing protocol emerged. This time each item on the list made perfect sense to me, even if it didn't make sense to anyone else.

It was entirely unprecedented to permit myself a) to have an opinion on a medical condition that differed from that of the experts and b) to follow through by acting on it.

I didn't always believe that what I was doing was going to bring me a child. Still I kept going back, pouring all my frustration and pain into action, choosing to doubt my doubt over and over again. I thought, if I don't conceive, at least I'll have the healthiest body I've ever had.

Eight months later I was pregnant.

Was it just luck? A coincidence? My diagnosis could've been a curse or a blessing. Rather than telling me I was "infertile," perhaps my elevated follicle stimulating hormone came to tell me I was far more fertile than I had ever allowed myself to be.

Does a holistic approach to health mean choosing acupuncture over in vitro fertilization? Or could it mean, as I and so many of my students have discovered, a choice between decisions based solely on statistics and other people's opinions, and action based on everything we know and discover about ourselves? When faced with a diagnosis, or a life crisis, do we turn a deaf ear to all the helpless voices inside us calling out for help, or give each one the attention it deserves? Do we perpetually search for someone to fight our battles, or learn what it takes to become our own fiercest allies?

Each time I speak to a group of women who yearn to become mothers, an image comes. From the corner of my eye I see a flock of cherry-cheeked babies streaming toward us, and each one of those babies is holding a parcel filled with gifts. Every once in a while a dimpled hand dips into a parcel and a gift tumbles through the clouds. For many of the women in that room, the work we do together will enhance the likelihood of a biological pregnancy. But the essence of the work is to pause, hold out our arms, and receive each gift as gracefully as we can.

Soon after my younger daughter, Adi, was born, I began to offer support to anyone who called for advice. Once *Inconceivable* was in print, strangers from around the world wrote to tell me they had emulated my process and now had miracles of their own. Others sought further guidance. Many were physicians, psychologists, lawyers, scientists, women with impressive credentials who had successfully navigated the world of academia, business, or medicine. Overnight, it seemed, these brilliant women had been reduced to little girls who sat around wringing their hands, waiting for instructions from the next Fertility Wizard. Many had been desperately revving up their ovaries with pharmaceuticals and invasive medical procedures, or half-heartedly pursuing a confusing array of natural treatments.

One late afternoon in May, the phone rang, and when I picked up the receiver, the woman on the other end of the line broke into sobs. "Sorry to call you out of the blue, " she said, catching her breath. "My name is Amy, and I just found your book at Barnes & Noble. My doctor left a message on my voice mail this morning and said I was in early menopause. I'm only thirty-three. He left a message on my voice mail! "

The following week I borrowed half a dozen folding

chairs from our next door neighbor, hunted down scattered scraps of paper with phone numbers, and invited everyone, including Amy, to our apartment on the Upper West Side of Manhattan for a Sunday afternoon.

Shortly before three o'clock the hallway was lined with shoes, a buzz of voices filled the living room, and the elevator continued to stop at our floor. Some women came with friends, and a few arrived with husbands who looked as though they were about to attempt their first high-wire act without a net.

There were not enough chairs, and we ended up sitting in a large circle on the floor. Perhaps it was the effect of the informal seating, or the fact that most of the people in the room had been sufficiently tenderized by years of frustration and grief, but not much time was wasted on small talk.

"I just can't get rid of this voice in the back of my head that says, You screwed up, you should've had a kid five years ago," said a small, delicate-featured woman. "But I couldn't, I wasn't ready, I would've resented the hell out of those kids. And I would've taken it out on Jeff," she added with a nervous laugh, sneaking a sidelong look at her handsome husband.

Amy spoke next. In a gray sweatshirt and jeans, her shiny, black cornrows pulled into a ponytail, she looked more like a college student than a high-powered lawyer. "My periods became excruciatingly painful when I was eighteen; I couldn't get through them without massive amounts of painkillers. Then my cousin said the Pill helped her. So I got a prescription, and it did help with the pain. But when I stopped taking it three years ago, things got worse than ever. "

Someone handed Amy a box of tissues, and a minute later an elegantly dressed redhead sitting near the window spoke.

"After the hysterosalpingogram, the doctor walked back into the room and said to the nurse : 'The tubes gotta go!' And he turned around and walked out. I swear I was thinking, Who is he talking to? Why is he talking about tire tubes?

"I let them do it. My fallopian tubes were clogged and they said I should have them out. And I let them do it." Her husband protectively put his arm around her shoulders. "We'll do whatever it takes, honey, whatever it takes!"

People sat motionless, listening carefully, as if something right around the corner, perhaps in what the next person might say, could be the key.

We began meeting regularly, and those Sunday afternoons eventually evolved into a series of workshops.

Initially the women who came to these gatherings had either been pronounced untreatable or had found themselves walking through the revolving doors of one fertility clinic after another. Yet even within this circle of statistical rejects, five out of seven people in one of the first groups were pregnant within six months. Three months after that initial phone call, Amy conceived her first child the old-fashioned way. Clearly, something I'd learned in the course of my own pilgrimage, which I was now sharing with others, was making a difference.

It seemed as though all my consciousness-raising adventures, the sense memory and movement work from my acting days, my lifelong fascination with wisdom traditions, every book I'd ever read, every poem I'd memorized as a child, had been a preparation for the task that was now before me. The various circumstances of the women who sought my help inspired new insights and additional exercises, and propelled the work far beyond the level I had originally intended.

After one of the meetings, Melody, a tall, striking brunette who had gone through five years of medical treatment, came up to me and said: "Finally, the truth!" What I think she meant was that the conversation that afternoon validated for Melody something she had long suspected: that there was a great deal more to discover about this challenge than what her lab reports revealed, and far more questions to be asked than those on the IVF clinic registration form.

For most of the women in our circle, the difficulty was not in their lack of willingness to make changes, or to recognize the many available options. The challenge, as I saw it, sprang from their belief that any advice worthy of attention had to come from an outside authority. The most frustrating aspect of this was that that voice of authority almost always reduced them to an age – or symptom – related statistic. Many of the natural healers would often emphasize one aspect of their difficulty and leave a large chunk of who these women were outside the examining room. As we worked together, first informally, then in a more structured setting, a sense of discovery gradually replaced despair. Seemingly small realizations began to add up.

"Do you know that I started buying books about infertility years before we even began trying? In *preparation* for trouble. It's crazy!!!"

"They told me this drug was going to trick my pituitary gland into producing less hormone. I'm thinking, why do I want to trick my pituitary; why can't my pituitary and I be on the same team?"

What brought the group together was the longing for a baby. But gradually, pregnancy became the side effect, not the primary goal of the work.

Jenna, a dreamy-eyed, petite brunette, attended one of my first workshops in New York City. As an art therapist, she worked with young adults in an outpatient clinic on

Long Island. She was in her early forties and didn't have a partner, so she'd decided to have a child on her own, using donor sperm. At some point during the session I asked everyone to answer the following question: "What is this baby going to bring you that you don't already have?" When Jenna's turn came, she burst into tears and said: "A new life, that's what I want! A new job, a new place to live, new people. I want a new life!"

After the workshop we spoke a couple of times, and then she disappeared. Three years later she called. It turned out that shortly after our session she'd decided to follow through on the insight that yes, she did want to be a mother, but she needed to get that new life first. Jenna accepted an assignment in Switzerland, met a man, and returned with him to the States. She was forty-five by then, and felt quite at peace with the idea of adoption. In spite of the barrage of discouraging statistics, she and her husband decided to give nature a chance before moving forward with a home study. The dark eyed little girl whose picture forms part of a collage hanging in my office is Jenna's daughter, conceived on the second try.

Celebrating my clients' pregnancies has been exciting. Equally or perhaps even more exciting has been witnessing the fact that everyone who's stayed the course has reclaimed her life in awe-inspiring ways. For the women who've chosen to adopt, the labor and the birth have been different than in biological pregnancies, but they have been equally thrilling and every bit as miraculous.

Perhaps one of my all-time favorite stories is the story of Ellen, a tall, statuesque investment banker, whose father was murdered when she was twelve. After being part of our circle for over a year, Ellen went on to adopt her daughter, Suzie. Here is one of her recent notes:

"Suzie will be 10 months next week. I can't believe it. We sing all the time. Whenever our 'family song' (I'm embarrassed to say, it's a top forty tune from Outkast) comes on – Suzie stops whatever she is doing, gets the biggest smile you've ever seen and starts singing. It would be impossible for me to love any child more than I love Suzie. Our work in the group has helped me in so many ways; after all the years of holding on to sadness, it made me feel free again. It opened up the world in a way I never imagined."

For me, the gift continues to unfold. After years of traveling and teaching seminars in a myriad of venues, I've often dreamed of building a space of our own, where people from different parts of the country could combine a day of learning with a full panoply of restorative adventures. When on our first visit to Woodstock one of the locals remarked that Woodstock is the place to find a really good pair of organic shoelaces, I knew we had hit gold. Set amid forested mountains, with great hiking trails, art galleries, spas, a raw foods deli, and a bakery with more varieties of organic breads than I can name, Woodstock turned out to be the perfect spot for the next chapter of the Fertile Heart story. After living on Manhattan's Upper West Side for almost thirty years, we became country folk in June 2001 and eventually built a small, comfortable space we call the Fertile Heart Studio. FHS, for short.

A couple of times a month I still travel to Manhattan to lead a support group. During my last trip to New York, I had lunch with Sarah, who once taught with me at Columbia University's American Language Program. I told her how rewarding it was to witness people who have been struggling with food addictions for years let go of lifelong habits within days. I told her about attending my first baptism, and other perks of my current job as a fertility educator.

Later that day, on the train ride back to Woodstock, I remembered something I hadn't thought about for years. As a schoolgirl in Czechoslovakia, during recess, I would go with the girls in my class to a nearby park to play circle games. In one game a child stood in the middle of the circle and chose a partner. The two children then clasped hands and spun round and round, while the rest of us sang and cheered them on. Usually by the time it was my turn to step into the center, recess was over.

Through the years I've often wondered why I felt like an outsider in those days. Though as an eight-year old child I could not have articulated this, being Jewish in a culture with a legacy of fierce anti-Semitism must've been part of it. And perhaps, feeling excluded, feeling "less than the rest" is something we all experience at one time or another. All I remember is that, more than anything else in the world, I longed to be as carefree and acceptable as I imagined everyone else to be.

Whenever I teach a workshop, part of me is back in the park with my exuberant classmates. Except now that small girl inside me is exactly like everyone else. An equal member of the circle, she gets to join the game, reach out her arms, and dance.

Chapter Two

Counting Snowflakes

"It is the intensity of the longing...
that does the work"

– Haleh Pourafzal and Roger Montgomery,
The Spiritual Wisdom of Hafez

The dove and the sparrow meet on their morning travels through the forest. "Tell me," asks the sparrow, "how much does a snowflake weigh?" "Why, nothing, snowflakes don't weigh anything" replies the dove.

"How is it then" asks the sparrow, "that as I sat this morning counting the snowflakes falling on the branch of the maple tree, when the six million seven hundred and third snowflake fell, the branch broke?"

– Tibetan tale

A soft spoken woman in a workshop once said, "I want this baby to fill up all the empty rooms in my house." The sadness and loss that accompanies us on this pilgrimage can be devastating. Yet at the center of our anguish is not the empty nursery, but the fear that it will remain empty forever. Part of us feels as though the baby market closed just minutes before we got there, and the child that was meant to be ours was handed over to someone else. How can we possibly let ourselves yearn for something that's unattainable?

Over the last fifteen years I've grown to have more trust in the wisdom that made me. I say, if there's longing, there's always the possibility of fulfillment. And if we're willing to keep walking – one way or another – we can get there from here.

Ɉot long ago, the American Society of Reproductive ͅ.ͧ.ͧ.ͧcine launched a public relations campaign to raise consciousness about our racing biological clocks. Their ad showed an upside-down baby bottle in the shape of an hourglass. At Fertile Heart we initiated our own counter-campaign. Instead of a baby bottle, our graphic featured an upside-down woman. Headstands are terrific for balancing our hormones. The idea of time as the great enemy is pervasive not only in the fertility world but in our culture in general, and it's a no-win game. Telling ourselves that we are falling behind schedule is hearing the roar of the fire-breathing dragon of self-blame. Choosing to feed this dragon or, as compassionately as we can, attempting to understand what it is that keeps us from moving forward in life is entirely up to us.

Last year while driving to a fertility conference in Connecticut, I passed a sign in the middle of the highway that said, "No Shortcuts to Anywhere Worth Going To." Since I'd spent so much of my life feeling trapped by my circumstances, I was always on the lookout for an all-purpose cosmic solution, a shortcut to nirvana, where whatever was amiss would be set right once and for all. Little by little I've come to surrender to the truth of that road sign. There really are no shortcuts.

The kindest thing people can do is assure you that setting out on a pilgrimage is an excellent idea. And if they can suggest a nifty compass, a tent, or a water filter that can save you from parasites, that's as good as it gets when it comes to helpful travel tips. To begin to view life as a mysterious unfolding, to surrender to the notion that whatever it is we're heading toward has its own time line, or that once we get there it may not look exactly the way it appears on the postcard (because the postcard couldn't do it justice), can save you much frustration. Better yet, it can allow you to appreciate the amazing scenery along the way.

Sophie, the spirited single woman I first met in one of the Woodstock workshops, could never have anticipated the inexplicable bond she felt with the two-year old girl who fell asleep nuzzling against her neck the moment the child was placed in her arms. "There were many children in the playroom where I first met my daughter, but as soon as I saw her face I knew this was my kid." This was not the way Sophie had once imagined becoming a mother. And yet she knew that what she was experiencing was as miraculous as any birth could have ever been. In the year I've known her, I've seen Sophie gather baskets upon baskets of berries along the trail that finally led to that small body leaning against her chest. The Sophie who traveled to Peru to bring her daughter home had a much larger view of her own life and her place in the world than the Sophie I'd met a year earlier.

After years of second-guessing my heart, I finally allowed myself to want a child more passionately than I'd ever wanted anything before. The face of the baby was the shiny apple I was willing to do anything in the world to reach, even if that meant giving up some of my most dearly held delusions. Etched in the far recesses of my psyche was a curious list of headings: Beware, each drop of happiness will cost you a bucket of suffering; You missed your chance, now you're too old to achieve anything of significance. On and on it went. But the pull of desire helped me unravel the truth. For someone who had been entangled in a web of such fabrications for decades, this was an unmistakable act of Grace.

Laura, an opera singer who flew to a Fertile Heart workshop in Woodstock from the West Coast, was reluctant to articulate just how deeply she wanted to be a mom.

"If I let myself feel it, it will hurt," she said.

"It's a little too late for that," I replied as gently as I could. "It already hurts. Not letting yourself feel the pain cuts off your emotional circulation. It stops life from moving through you."

Laura's question comes up in just about every workshop. It's a question I ask myself every time I'm about to tackle a new challenge:

Do I really want to make myself that vulnerable, and give that much of myself again? .

Most of the time, I'd rather stay put. I'm scared of being misunderstood, of appearing foolish. But the truth is, I don't really have a choice. Because the real question Laura and I are wrestling with is: How much of a human experience am I willing to have this time around? How alive do I dare to be?

If I really worked at it, I could spend the rest of my time on earth feeling as little as possible. Then maybe I could keep out of harm's way, and make it safely all the way to my grave. I'd get to have "a Near-Life Experience," which is what so many of us settle for.

The idea, of course, is to translate everything – the yearning, the pain and the joy, the rage and the passion – into some form of useful, consistent action. If a doctor were to put us on a course of antibiotics, chances are we'd take them every day. Similarly, for any action to become medicine, we need to *treat* it as medicine. And that takes discipline, a word which has somehow gotten a bad rap in our culture, implying as it often does, self-sacrifice or even punishment: doing the right thing even if it kills us. The word "discipline" has the same root as "disciple," which means student. For me, discipline has to do with learning something. And learning is meant to be a highly pleasurable activity. So, perhaps to be truly disciplined means to cultivate a kind of patience with ourselves, to take ourselves by the hand and say, "Come, this is the trail we're gonna follow." And to whenever we're tempted to wander off, take ourselves by the hand over and over again. Gently. Lovingly. It means showing in our behavior that we are militantly on our own side.

What I usually witness with clients who stay the course is that the pleasure of discovery and learning intensifies as they deepen their commitment to regular practice.

Years ago, I heard these lines from a poem by Yehuda Halevi, an eleventh century mystic, and they instantly changed the way I thought about my various pursuits:

> *I sought your nearness with all my heart,*
> *I called you and going out to meet you*
> *I found you coming toward me.*

If we keep putting one foot in front of the other, one day we discover that our child has been walking toward us all along.

Trust it, and our baby-longing can become the golden rope we hold on to as we ascend the slippery cliffs of our fears. Each sip of vegetable juice, each imagery exercise, each meeting at the adoption agency is a snowflake that adds weight to our efforts. Our evolving healing regimen is the friend we turn to on days when the voice of futility threatens to drown out all other sounds. On those days, and especially on those days, we remind ourselves of the sparrow and the dove, and unroll our yoga blanket, pick up a dream journal, or do whatever it takes to climb out of bed. Unless, of course, staying in bed and pulling up the covers is what the situation calls for.

As Mary Oliver writes in a poem called "West Wind":

There is life without love.
It is not worth a bent penny or a scuffed shoe.

So, I say, there is nothing better you can do than to lean into the ache and row, row toward the life you once imagined. And don't stop rowing till you get there. Buy a copy of *Winnie the Pooh*, inscribe it to your child, and read it out loud to someone you love. Trust that it will one day be your son's favorite bedtime story. Doing this will make the juices of life flow through you more freely. And it might even work a miracle on your cervical mucus.

Let your yearning be the compass that keeps you on course. Let it be the tent that shelters you through the harshest storm, the water filter that screens out fear and keeps you hydrated with hope. Gather your snowflakes. When the time comes, the branch will break.

Chapter Three

The Authority Vested in You

"In a novel everything seems so simple. But when you yourself are in love, you realize that no one knows anything, that each has to decide for himself."

– Anton Chekhov, *The Three Sisters*

When God created human beings, the angels were jealous because God had endowed the humans with divine wisdom that would guide them through life. So the jealous angels conspired to hide this gift from the humans. "Let's take it to the peak of the highest mountain," said one. "No," said another, "Let's bury it at the bottom of the deepest sea." But the smartest angel of all said: "Let's hide divine wisdom deep inside each person. It's the last place they'll ever look."

— Hasidic legend

The hint of hope that led me to question medical certainty came from a voice deep inside me, one that had been straining to rise up for as long as I can remember.

The one-party regime of Communist Czechoslovakia did not favor listening to inner truth. The job ahead was clear: Communism, the saving grace of mankind, promised a just world for all. Each of us was called upon to use our talents to help turn this grand vision into reality.

For me, the assignment came rather early. In second grade my teacher, Mrs. Novak, asked me to participate in a nation wide poetry reading contest. I came in second in the region, which, according to Mrs. Novak, was a splendid achievement.

From then on I took my place as one of the official school orators at the May Day parade, on the anniversary of the

Russian Revolution, and at other state-mandated celebrations.

Each year on International Women's Day, clad in my young Communist uniform (pleated navy blue skirt, crisp white blouse, a red kerchief tied around my neck), I rode the bus to the county fair in the nearest village to deliver a poem befitting the occasion. Once, as I was about to announce the title, someone in the last row called out: "We can't see anything back here!" A pair of hands lifted me up on a milk crate and there I stood, feeling tall and powerful, pouring my passion into the grandiose lines.

> *We're marching, marching,*
> *Soldiers of a most unusual army,*
> *Army of peace,*
> *That declares war on war!*

The room broke into tumultuous applause, and afterward the peasant women of the village cooperative pinched my cheeks and patted my head. *To je nasha dievchinka!* "She's our girl!" they said, squeezing a fresh baked bun into my hands.

I loved being seen and heard, and missing days of school to travel around the country with a group of adults. But my special assignment didn't require independent thinking or decision-making. I had no access to anything more substantial than the propaganda poems of the day, and even if I had, the choice of material was strictly controlled by party officials.

Had I not left Czechoslovakia a year after the Russian invasion in 1969, I might've spent much of my adult life as an official orator of my homeland.

Although most of the people who have participated in the Fertile Heart work grew up in a political climate quite different from mine, the art of self-reliance was not on the syllabuses of their graduate programs. Helene, a small woman with short brown layered hair came up to me one day after a workshop. "You know," she said, her cheeks flushed with the afternoon's revelations. "I realized today that with all my fancy degrees, no one has ever taught me to believe in myself."

Now the stakes were high, and each decision felt like a life-and-death choice:

"I've gone to three different clinics and every doctor tells me to move right to IVF, and to hike up my meds, but a woman I know just conceived with minimal stimulation. What if this is my last chance and I blow it?"

The first thing I say is that every decision you make takes you one step closer to your child. Each outcome, however disappointing, becomes the next guidepost. And if you learn to use your inner resources and begin to see each action as the next stop on a pilgrimage, "blowing it" is simply not within the realm of possibility.

At one time or another, every one of us hopes to be saved. We hope the next e-mail, the next message on our voice mail will bring the cure for whatever ails us. Over and over I receive letters from readers looking for a weekly meal plan or some other formula to follow. For every person convinced that a formula, a diet, a pill, or an herb was what got them pregnant, there are ten women who've tried the very same fix and walked away empty-handed. That doesn't mean that the books and workshops that offer formulas are useless. But if we adapt any of them without doing our own experimentation and research, we pay a price.

Lori, a physical therapist with a busy practice and an aging mom who'd recently moved into Lori's Manhattan apartment, had suffered from endometriosis most of her life. When I met her she was following a diet outlined by a popular self-help book. The author advised women who suffered from this condition to eliminate dairy and replace it with soy. Lori went on a processed soy safari, and her endometriosis became more painful than ever. When I suggested that she rethink this choice, she began an investigation that led to a more thoughtful approach to working with food, and her symptoms eventually subsided. The healing of Lori's endometriosis became a much more demanding, but also more mysterious and exciting, assignment than she'd ever imagined.

In the fall of 2004, I began leading a twice-monthly phone support circle. On Sunday evening at eight o'clock, women and a few courageous husbands call in to practice the tools they'd learned in the workshop, or simply to find out more about the Fertile Heart work.

"I've been seeing a great healer. I mean she's supposed to be amazing, but I really can't tell if I'm getting anything out of it," Annie, a Minneapolis lawyer, remarked as we began our session.

"What does she do?" I asked.

"She makes sounds. She puts her hands on my stomach and belts out an *aaaaaah*."

"Why does she do that?" queried another voice on the line.

"She says she's connecting with the soul of the baby."

"What about you? What do you do while this is going on? Do you feel you're connecting with your baby when she does that?" I asked.

"Usually I end up dozing. I see her after work: I'm pretty wiped out," Annie replied.

Now, I'm a great believer in working with sound. A deep sigh, a growl, or a scream can be good medicine. The voice is a wondrous tool that can bring to the surface what is hidden inside us, and anything that helps clear away some of the inner clutter carves out more space for conception. Though I'm sure that Annie's healer was using sound for the right reasons, Annie was left out of the process. She was handing herself entirely over to the healer and her reputation.

The temptation to let someone else do our thinking for us is huge. Perhaps because most of us didn't get as much caretaking as we would've liked, we keep hoping to find the one person who will finally give us everything we need. But a child in us also cries, "Myself! I can do it myself!" That child wants to grow up, to live her own life, to wrestle with choices, and to choose her next move without supervision. That child knows instinctively that taking risks is the most exciting piece of being alive, that otherwise we all might as well go through our daily routine, turn on the TV every night, and slowly slip into a collective coma.

Engaging consultants, whether they be physicians or acupuncturists or therapists, can be eminently useful as long as you don't see them as anything more than your esteemed consultants and you don't leave yourself out of the equation. The word "doctor" means "teacher." In the best of all worlds the task of these helpers is to teach you to read your symptoms, to help you understand the workings of the remedies they offer, and to show you how to collaborate with the intelligence of your body. Their task is to encourage self- trust.

As Ralph Waldo Emerson wrote, "What lies behind us and what lies ahead of us are tiny matters compared to what lies within us." Since it is *within* you, it is pretty much hidden from everyone else's view. Though your best friend or teacher might sense your talents, the only magician that can reach in and pull out one shiny scarf of creation after another is you. And if you continue to reach in, what you draw forth will never cease to astound you.

So how do we learn to intrinsically trust ourselves

when for as long as we can remember we've been taught that – mother, father, teacher, priest, doctor – knows better than we do. Where do we look for the courage to say, "I don't think so; no, that doesn't make any sense to me." Or to listen politely to the views of our advisors, feign a quick look at the clock, mutter an apology, and make a beeline for the exit.

In one of my treasured companion books, *Letters to a Young Poet*, Rainer Maria Rilke gives pretty clear directions on connecting with inner knowing: "Nobody can counsel and help you, nobody. There is only one single way. Go into yourself."

Most of us tend not to "go into ourselves" until we have gone everywhere else, getting a second, third, and umpteenth opinion, and still finding ourselves clueless about our next move. A friend of mine calls this "fiddling with the dial" rather than waiting for the reception to clear.

Standing still for a while – resisting the urge to sprint into a marathon phone session with our advisor – can get us over the first hurdle. So when my clients tell me about their best friend who conceived on her fifth in vitro cycle, and a neighbor who's adopting, or their aunt Sally who's sending them articles on donor eggs, I remind them of the Chinese book of wisdom, the Tao Te Ching, which asks: "Do you have the patience to wait till your mud settles and the water is clear? Can you remain unmoving till the right action arrives all by itself?"

This inner voice may rise up unexpectedly, from a line in a poem, a fragment of overheard conversation, a shiver that runs through you as you listen to someone's story. At first this voice might be no more than a barely audible whisper, a small bird singing in your head. But learning how to feed this bird, and engaging in activities that make her sing out with more confidence, can keep you sane. It can help you unearth a hidden archive of images and memories. In this archive all of your life's events, large and small, traumatic and joyful, are meticulously recorded. As you search through the documents, you begin to understand the heart of your ambitions and desires. And before long you find yourself immersed in the most challenging and the most exciting research project of your life, in which you are the lab, the subject of the experiment, and the chief scientist and decision maker. Everything you have ever learned and experienced is put to exquisite use.

Over and over again, I witness a major shift in attitude whenever a client begins to contact this place of inner certainty.

In the spring of 1998, Cynthia and her husband, Charles, sat in the first row of my workshop at the Learning Annex in New York. I was moved by the grief on Cynthia's face and the way she held on to her husband's hand. They looked so young. I remember thinking that she must've been given a pretty hopeless prognosis to be so devastated. It turned out that Cynthia was thirty-two, but since she hadn't responded well to several stimulated cycles, her doctor had suggested that she might be going through early menopause. "He told me he was willing to try one in vitro cycle, but that I should seriously start thinking about a donor egg," said Cynthia, tears streaming down her face.

Perhaps with Cynthia, as with me, desperation inspired a swift and solid connection with her own truth. Soon the certainty with which she began making her decisions were clearly arising out of a deep inner knowing. After the workshop she began to record her dreams, practice imagery, and considerably lighten her workload.

During an imagery exercise, Cynthia realized that one of the reasons she longed for a biological child was the fact that she had lost both of her parents at a very young age and spent her childhood ~~being shipped~~ from one aunt to another. "It's my chance to see what it's like to have a real family," she said. That insight brought old grief to the surface, but it also gave her the courage to stop all treatment, including monitoring of her hormone levels.

She was still in touch with a number of women she met at the fertility clinic. "They think I've completely lost my mind, and they're telling me this holistic hand-holding is costing me precious time, but I just know, right now, that is what I have to do," she told us one day as she unrolled a 20-by-40 inch canvas. "I came home from work and took out my watercolors. I haven't done that in ages. "

The bold, generous curves and vibrant colors spoke more eloquently about Cynthia's fertility than a battery of hormone tests ever could.

Cynthia followed her own truth with growing confidence. Her daughter, Lilli, was conceived sooner than any of us expected, and when Lilli was eleven months old, Cynthia called to tell me she was pregnant again.

The struggle to trust ourselves doesn't necessarily stop after we've won our first battle. Sometimes, the frightened child within us finds herself in a brand-new place and panics. "Now you've done it," she says. "This is not the way good girls behave. Now daddy, mommy, teacher, doctor will not love you anymore."

Last September I got an e-mail from Emma, a client I had worked with a year earlier.

Hi Julia,

Thank God, my pregnancy has been going quite smoothly. But I did have an episode last week that I wonder about. On Wednesday morning I had been sitting at my desk and suddenly I felt very hot. I got up to splash some water on my face and thought I was going to faint. Somehow I made it back to my desk and after a while I was okay again. When I called my doctor he said not to worry, that pregnant women are susceptible to heat. But when I thought about the timing, I realized that one year ago, almost to the minute, I had taken the blood test that showed my elevated hormone levels. Just a couple of days prior to this episode, Scott and I talked about this "anniversary" coming up and how incredible it was that things have turned out the way they did.

I am thinking that perhaps my body made the connection with that date of one year ago. I was trying to think what you would suggest and I came up with an imagery exercise. In the exercise I flushed last year's test results down the drain, and I invited an image of peace and serenity to move through my body.

Emma was standing up for herself with this pregnancy in a way she had never done before, aligning herself with an authority far greater than the authority of statistics. But part of her was not entirely sure that this was permissible behavior. She invented her own imagery exercise to work through the doubt, and the rest of her pregnancy was quite uneventful. On the first day of spring, Emma delivered a robust baby boy.

When I first came to America, I lived with my aunt Lillian, and each evening we sat spellbound watching her favorite TV show, *To Tell the Truth*. Three contestants, all claiming to be the same person, tell the audience their name, say, Dr. Dolittle. A panel of celebrities tries to figure out who the two impostors are by asking a series of questions. At a climactic moment, the host calls out: "Will the real Dr. Dolittle please stand up?" All three contestants shift in their chairs, and finally the real one rises.

This voice of "inner certainty" is the part of us that continues to cry out: "Will the real Julia, Debbie, Susan please stand up?" At crossroads, what terrifies us is not that we will make a mistake. What terrifies us is that our lives will turn into an endless game show, and the person we know to be our most genuine self will never get the chance to stand up.

The good news is that each time we recognize the truth and act on it even in the smallest way – "No, I'm not ready for my next in vitro;" "Wheatgrass juice is not my thing;" Please, Doctor, telling me I have the ovaries of a sixty-year old is not a very helpful way to deliver your diagnosis" – we find ourselves breathing a little more freely.

"By the authority vested in me." What a wonderful phrase! Each time we make our doctors or our advisors into gods that will answer all our prayers, a portion of the Authority naturally conferred on us is lost. In such a transaction we are not the only injured party. The person we idolize is seduced into feeling that he has more power than he truly does, and is therefore robbed of the delights of life-long learning.

Many times in the last ten years, something has opened up in the person I've been working with and I experienced a deep knowing that conception was not far away. But I would have never dared to interrupt the woman's revelatory process. Telling you a pregnancy ought to be possible is one thing, but prophesizing it is quite another. Countless times women have told me that a healer has suggested that if they follow his advice, they will be pregnant in four months. When they're not, they're angry. If doctors or healers volunteer such a prediction, they're handing you something that is not theirs to give.

Ironically, our own truest voice cannot rise up without humility. We have to give up our need to be right; we need to be willing to receive life as a series of sacred instructions from the kindest of invisible Teachers. This is something I wrestle with only about a hundred times a day. But the struggle is worth it. Because, after all these years, I have learned beyond any doubt that the more willingly I bow to this Teacher within me, the less I suffer.

Part Two

The Human Loaf

Chapter 4

The Unbearable Oneness of Being

"You can feed her all day with the vitamin A
and the Bromofiz, but the medicine never
gets anywhere near where the trouble is."

– Frank Loesser, *Guys and Dolls*

Naaman is a captain in the army of the king of Aram, and a leper. One day his servant says: "Master, I heard of a man in a far-off land, a healer. Elisha is his name. You must see him." Naaman sets off on a journey loaded down with ten talents of silver and six thousand pieces of gold. Surely, he thinks, getting healed from such a dreadful disease will be a costly affair. When Naaman comes before the healer, he is told to wash seven times in the River Jordan. "How dare you insult me with such foolishness!" responds Naaman. "Aren't you going to mix a brew, or smooth a salve over my flesh? If bathing is all it takes, surely the rivers of my own land are as good as yours."

"Master," whispers the servant, "what's there to lose?" So Naaman swallows his pride and lowers his body into the River Jordan seven times. And lo and behold, when he steps out of the water his flesh is as smooth and soft as silk.

– Adapted from Kings 5:1-14

When I was in graduate school, finishing my master's in teaching, one of my professors used to say: "In the classroom there is nothing like a good prop, especially if the students get to eat it after it has served its purpose."

The prop I like to use is a loaf of organic, multigrain, freshly baked bread. I hold it up and ask, "Can you name some of the ingredients?"

"Yeast, flour, water," my students call out.

Then I break off a piece, and continue. "And how about this? What ingredients are present here?"

"The same." We conclude that even the tiniest crumb contains all of the ingredients.

"What if I change something in the mix, say, add a little more water?" I ask. No one seems to doubt that every morsel of the loaf will reflect the change.

Wouldn't the same hold true for the Holy Human Loaf? A mix of flesh, intellect, mystery, and passion? Doesn't it make sense that here too, the smallest change in the batter – a flash of insight, a disparaging remark, a flicker of hope – will affect every atom we're made of? In spite of the growing body of scientific literature on the biochemical effect of beliefs, in spite of decades of the emotional detox many of us have endured with our various therapists, in spite of the cathedrals we've built to honor the Mystery pulsing through us, when a symptom shows up we, like Naaman, look for brews or salves to make us well. Somehow we think that if we tinker with our hormones long enough, the numbers will line up and our bodies will perform as instructed.

Next time you sense a volcano of rage lift you out of your chair, or feel a wave of gratitude wash over you, stop and observe your breath. See if you can let go of the story for a few seconds and just sense the current of energy generated within you. Is it possible that what you're experiencing isn't having physiological consequences? That although the trigger was not physical, not even a single cell in your body is detached from the experience? This is not trigonometry. It should not require extensive training to observe the answers to these questions in your own body or in another's.

Just watch your best friend turn beet red when the man she's been telling you about enters the room.

One of the great revelations for me in these last fifteen years has been seeing just how much our feelings and the yearning of the soul is mirrored in our biology: how eloquently the body speaks of everything we try to keep hidden from ourselves and the world.

"Life is a mystery to be lived, not a problem to be solved," said the philosopher Soren Kirkegaard. When we bring the idea of this Oneness of Being into our daily, laundry-and-dishes consciousness, we get closer to Kirkegaard's notion of seeing our difficulties as mysteries to be lived; mysteries which continually call us to be more intimate with ourselves, each other, and the world. We begin to see our difficulties as mysteries to be lived and put to good use, rather than problems to be solved and be done with, or worse yet some sort of karmic punishment to be endured.

What else can each task set before us be if not an invitation to understand this Oneness more and more deeply? I can't say this principle is easy to adhere to in my own life. But I keep opening myself up to it a little more each day. The alternative of feeling unlucky or undeserving or powerless is simply no longer an option.

Lucy, a woman with honey-colored hair and a round, open face, was sitting directly in my line of vision at a lecture I gave in Chicago some years ago. As I spoke I watched her eyes grow more alert, her mouth slowly widen into a smile, her body lean forward in anticipation. At some point toward the end of the session she sighed out loud and said: "God, this sounds too good to be true, but it makes a lot of sense!"

She stayed in touch with me for the next four months via phone and e-mail. During that time, Lucy began to challenge her lifestyle, rethink a good many of her beliefs, and draw a great deal of strength from her family's rich tradition of Irish folk wisdom. When she called to tell me the news of her pregnancy, she said, "Remember that talk you gave at the conference? You said your baby journey was the first time you really followed through on something. I decided to go for broke. You know how professional athletes, when they ask them if they would change anything about the game, say, 'I left it all on the court,' meaning they did all they could do? Well, that's what I decided I was gonna do. In this game I was gonna leave it all on the court. It was like some switch got thrown inside me. I could feel it."

When a magazine reporter called a year later and asked for a testimonial about my work, I asked Lucy if she'd be willing to share her story. "Sure, I love talking about it," she said.

But when the reporter e-mailed me the story, it was quite different from the one I had witnessed. Mainly it was a tale of the mechanics of Lucy's acupuncture sessions and a list of her vitamin supplements. There was no mention of the work she had done revising her beliefs and opening up the neural pathways so that the medicine could *get* to where the trouble was. All of that was forgotten.

Fifteen months later I heard from Lucy again. She was desperately trying to give her son Benjamin a baby brother, and this time neither the acupuncture nor a medicine cabinet filled with vitamins were doing the trick. Why? Perhaps because the ever-changing, Holy Human Loaf called Lucy was not the same loaf she had been three years earlier. It was time to begin again, and to set out in search of images and clues, sensations and revelations to point the way.

When we are lured into thinking that this or that thing will do it for us, that all we need to do is do yoga every day, or meditate, or drink wheatgrass, we leave out the most essential piece of any practice and sometimes do more harm than good. We reinforce the false notion that we are less than a miracle.

A beloved teacher and scholar, Arthur Green, tells a story of a bookstore in Berkeley during the sixties with a sign over the entrance that read something like this:

> *Scientology Doesn't Work.*
> *Transcendental Meditation Doesn't Work.*
> *Chanting Doesn't work.*
> *Yoga Doesn't Work.*
> *You Work!*

The only practice that will do it for us is one we can engage in with every fiber of our being: a practice we deepen and reinvent over and over again. A practice we can live as if our life depended on it.

Soon after her second child, another strapping boy, was born, Lucy and I discussed this idea of, as she put it, "fessing up" that so much of our lives has to do with our choices.

"If I just said it was the acupuncture and the vitamins that did it for me, I was off the hook, but if I had something to do with it, not getting pregnant meant I failed; it was my fault."

When your mind tunes into radio YSKB (You Should've Known Better), you have a choice of turning up the volume or changing the station. The tools and ideas I share in this book were the golden rope I hung on to when there was little else I could do. The thing about a golden rope is that you can use it to climb up to heaven or you can tie it into a noose.

Yes, we are co-creators of our lives, but co-creators only. Saying that our actions can make a difference doesn't mean we're omnipotent. Our lives have been shaped by countless forces, and we, each of us, always do the best we can. So, to paraphrase a famous line of Winston Churchill's: Never, Never, Never, Never, Never blame yourself. Never! You'd be giving yourself too much credit. Besides, it's a huge waste of natural resources, namely your time, your talents, and your life force. No matter what real or perceived errors we've committed over the years, the good news is that with each breath we can begin again.

One other thing that helps me see how I nail down the hardwoods and hinge the doors of this house called my life is paying attention to the words I use.

We create by naming things.

We see a number on a lab report and we name it. Premature Ovarian Failure, Hostile Mucus, Incompetent Cervix, Poor Responder. We then flap that name at the person like a hat, leave out the seventeen thousand variables that make them who they are, and create them in our own image. Depending on how powerful we appear in the eyes of the person we name, she can either accept our vision as fact or ignore it as best she can.

The mouth is the gateway between the inner and outer world. That which crosses to the other side reveals us startlingly to ourselves as the most impressionable of creatures. We may find that we've unwittingly ingested other people's beliefs the way one absentmindedly swallows an hors d'oeuvre at a cocktail party.

"Our insurance *only* pays for three IVF cycles, and I was told with my numbers I might not even be a *candidate* for ART," lamented Amelia at one of our twice-monthly phone support circles.

"It sounds like you're running for office, and you don't have the budget for a decent campaign, and even if you did, the elections are rigged, " I suggested lightly.

"That's exactly what it feels like," said Amelia.

"I know, but it's a feeling, just a feeling," someone else said. "I'm beginning to realize I can only walk toward this baby one step at a time, and it works a lot better when I do that. When I start freaking out, I keep reminding myself that by the time I'll get to point B, I might know something I couldn't know today. But I have to live my way to that point. I guess I've given up wanting to control everything all the time."

When it comes to healing, I often think about the three little words whose utterance might induce droves of people to set out in search of more satisfying answers.

"I don't know."

What if the expert you turned to said, "I don't know. I don't know how to help you. This is the only thing I can offer for now. If you find out anything more, please come back and tell me."

An interesting term often crops up in the medical terminology of reproductive difficulties. When no readily identifiable diagnosis exists, either structural or hormonal, aspiring mothers and fathers are told they have "unexplained infertility" As if the creation of life on any level, whether a fully functioning kidney or a regular heartbeat, is ever fully explainable.

In 2001, a few weeks before the World Trade Center tragedy, I interviewed Dr. Zev Rosenwaks, director of the Center for Reproductive Medicine and Infertility at the New York Presbyterian Hospital.

"With some couples, everything in their diagnostic work-up checks out, and the cycle fails. Then I see women with all the cards stacked against them, and they end up with a healthy baby. Even in the best of circumstances we have no more than a sixty percent marker of viability. In other words, there is a lot about this that's quite beyond us."

Sadly, this kind of humility rarely reaches the consulting

rooms.

Peter, a tall, imposing-looking man with a high forehead and a good-natured laugh, spoke about this at a recent workshop:

"When we did our first in vitro, our doctor himself called and asked that we both get on the phone. 'We did it!' he said. 'I think we got that last good egg just in time, the numbers look great, congratulations!'

"At seven weeks, a day after we saw the heartbeat, the nurse left a message telling us the numbers didn't look good. When Catherine went in for the D & C..."

Peter's voice trailed off, and he looked down at his hands, "And ...the doctor told us he didn't know what happened. He said, 'It's not like there is something we could've done to prevent it.'

"The pregnancy was their doing, but not the miscarriage."

To borrow the perfect words of theologian Abraham Joshua Heschel: "How embarrassing for man to be the greatest miracle on earth and not to understand it." I'm certain that somewhere near the floor of the soul, underneath our terror and our need to be right, we do sense the Mystery and yearn to understand it. No backdrops bring forth the Unbearable Oneness of flesh, intellect, heart, and soul as startlingly as the world of baby making.

There may be hidden reasons why our bodies behave as they do, and there are many we can learn to decode. We'd certainly be foolish not to try. If the body can't handle the workload, or if it's the heart that's frightened, or the soul that wishes to soar, we must stop, pull up a chair, and find out what the trouble is. Otherwise we can blast our ovaries with stimulants, produce caravans of embryos of the highest grade, and still go home to an empty nursery.

Chapter 5

Image by Image

"...the most remarkable feature of imagery work is that it can be accompanied by physiological changes."

– Gerald Epstein, M.D., *Healing Visualizations*

*T**he ancient Greeks sometimes built a small temple for Apollo at a crossroads. If someone didn't know which road to take, he or she could go inside the temple, meditate in silence, and find out which way to go.*

– Greek folklore

In an acting class devoted to Greek theater, I first heard about Apollo's temple. "We humans are always grappling with choices; much of the time we're split, and where two roads intersect inside us no one has built a temple," my professor would say as we analyzed the motivation of each character. Whether we are facing a life-threatening diagnosis or a day at the laundromat, life is a never-ending flow of decision-making. In my own growth as well as that of my students, imagery practice has become an extraordinary tool for kneading the Human Loaf and building an inner sanctuary, a space we can enter when we're not sure which path to take. Sometimes a thirty-second exercise is all that is needed for the answer to rise up:

See yourself at a fork in the road. Take one step in one direction and keep walking. How do you feel? Is there anyone else around? Observe the vegetation, the weather, the color of the sky. Do you wish to continue walking in this direction?

> *Breathe out once and return to the fork in the*
> *road. Do you wish to try the alternate route? If*
> *so, begin walking and observe your experience.*
> *Repeat the exercise each day until the choice of*
> *paths is clear.*

Although I could not have named it at the time, my first deliberate practice of imagery began when I was eight years old. Our family lived in a small house in Kosice, a town in the eastern part of Czechoslovakia. Only one of the rooms was heated during the long winters, and the four of us – my mother, father, sister, and I – slept, ate, argued, and generally carried on with our lives in that one room. It was not the calmest of living quarters. I wrestled with countless disturbing feelings in those days, and often had trouble settling into sleep. Counting sheep didn't work, nor did a number of other strategies, but one day an idea came.

After climbing into bed that night, I closed my eyes and conjured up pictures, one frame for each member of my family. I would see my older sister handing me a snack, my mother with her arms open for a hug. I found great solace in my secret slide show. The images calmed me, connected me with my love for my parents and sister, and erased uncomfortable residues left over from the day. If I fought a lot with my sister, I would do extra footage of her performing good deeds. To this day, I'm grateful to that eight-year-old inside me for knowing where to turn for an antidote to the constant chaos and tension around her.

In my twenties and thirties, I used various forms of imagery, mostly as a relaxation tool, a "Close your eyes, and listen to the waves," kind of thing. The thought of using it as a treatment option for a hopeless diagnosis seemed a little far-fetched. I had much more faith in sharp instruments – like a needle and a syringe full of stimulants – than in the power of my imagination. But since needles and syringes were not an option, I put skepticism on hold and took my daily dose of imagery medicine as one would follow a course of antibiotics. Gradually the experience of the images became more and more real. Not only that, my body seemed to be responding with sensations, feelings, and insights.

I share this with you because what's important initially is a commitment to regular practice. As my friend Lowell, a former Jesuit monk, likes to say: "To wait for faith in order to be able to pray is putting the cart before the horse." Your belief will emerge from the practice.

One of my early teachers, the psychiatrist Gerald Epstein, often discussed the exciting physiological changes induced by mental imagery. He argued that since Western medicine accepted the idea that shifts in our body chemistry can affect the way we feel and think, and how we see the world (through antidepressants, for example), why should it be so difficult to believe the reverse? The images we live with have biological consequences. Just think of how many times you've woken up from a nightmare drenched in sweat, your heart racing. Yet when you opened your eyes, there was no one there; the changes in your heart rate and the beads of sweat on your forehead had been triggered by a series of pictures.

Some years ago, Dr. Ellen Langer, author and professor of psychology at Harvard Medical School, told me about a study that illustrated this beautifully. In 1985, Dr. Langer placed an advertisement in a Boston newspaper, asking for volunteers over the age of seventy to participate in an experiment. She took them all to a retreat outside of Boston, where they played a game for ten days. The object of the game was for all of the one hundred volunteers to pretend that they were living in the 1950s. They were told to just be who they were thirty years ago. To help make the game as real as possible, the entire retreat was structured in the style of the 50s: music, furniture, movies, magazines, fashion, the news. Everyone discussed the kitchen debates of Khrushchev and Nixon and the politics of Fidel Castro in the present tense.

After ten days, Dr. Langer measured a number of biological markers, such as physical strength, hearing, vision, hand grip, finger length, weight, and height, and compared them with the measurements that were taken at the beginning of the study. Amazingly, she found that ten days of collective change in the perception of these people resulted in a reversal of biological aging by several years. A significant number of the volunteers grew in height. Joint flexibility and finger length increased. Many could hear and see better. Independent judges, who looked at photographs at the beginning and the end of the study, estimated that after the experiment the volunteers looked, on average, three years younger. (Dr. Langer describes this and other fascinating experiments in her book *Mindfulness*)

I cite this study to show clients how important it is not to be sucked into the collective belief of "aging eggs" and statistics. That kind of thinking sets you up for failure before you even begin trying.

Much of the time, physicians and caregivers don't realize the enormous power of the words they use. A couple of years ago, Beth, a client undergoing IVF treatment, sent me the following e-mail: "You won't believe this," she wrote, "but in the middle of the embryo transfer my doctor said he wanted to be sure I knew that I had no more than a five percent chance of this working. He said he wanted to spare me from disappointment. He might've meant well, but boy his timing was off. Too late for that, Doc! I wanted to say. Then I remembered the golden shield exercise we did in group. So I closed my eyes, took a deep breath, and watched those words bounce right off my shield. I don't think any of them got anywhere near those tiny embryos. " It turned out Beth's embryos either didn't hear that the odds were against them or just didn't care, because I have a picture of two little boys who showed up nine months later.

For most of us, the images that control our daily lives are automatic. The programming for them was installed long ago. Sometimes that early programming makes us stumble through life as if we were following the posthypnotic suggestions of our worst enemies. The Fertile Heart imagery practice uses pictures the way a diviner aims a divining rod. The right image called up at an appropriate time jolts the memory and points to the exact place inside us where the life force is trying to break through the rocks of fear.

Last year I worked with Samantha, a woman in her early forties. In the middle of our first phone call, she sighed despairingly, "How can I ever expect to have a baby, when I can't even imagine myself being pregnant? I never could. I was talking to an old friend the other day – we've known each other since junior high – and she reminded me how I would always space out when someone started talking about having babies."

I suggested the following exercise to Samantha as part of her self-healing protocol for the next fourteen days.

See yourself standing in the Room of Fear. What are the images, people, and objects you see and sense in this room? Breathe out once and look around. Face that which frightens and worries you. Now turn to your right and find the exit, the doorway to freedom. Open this door and step outside. Know that the images in this room provide the next clue; they are here to teach you something. And know that you can always find your way out of the Room of Fear.

Samantha reported later that the walls of the Room of Fear were lined with empty bookshelves. After we talked for a while, it turned out that as a young girl, Samantha used to visit her aunt, a gynecologist, who often shared with her stories of patients. She learned of miscarriages, abortions, and other assorted baby troubles, complete with graphics from the many textbooks that lined the walls of her aunt's study.

"Sometimes I would be sick to my stomach after those visits, and I remember thinking there was probably something wrong with me, too," said Samantha. "That all those things could happen to me. And then at eighteen my periods became irregular and my aunt said I should just go on the Pill, that she had many patients who did that and that eventually my cycles would straighten themselves out. But they never did."

Trapped inside Samantha was a ten-year-old girl horrified by the pictures in her aunt's books. But next to that girl was also a young woman longing for a baby, wondering what it would feel like to be a mom. Several months of work engaged these two hidden parts of Samantha and repaired the destructive influence of those early impressions. For the first time in her life, she began to see herself with a round swollen belly, and she began having dreams of being pregnant. Curiously, it seemed everyone around her was suddenly announcing their first pregnancies. But this time, the news was less a threat than a message of encouragement, as if the universe was saying, "See? It can be done!" A few weeks later, on a rainy Wednesday afternoon, Samantha called to share the news: She was pregnant.

Rilke's story "Of One Who Listened to the Stones" describes how Michelangelo was able to listen with his hands and feel figures trapped in a block of marble, a shoulder here, a pair of trembling hands there. How he felt that they had been there all along. As he chiseled away the excess stone, he freed them and lifted them out of the rock.

Etched bone-deep inside us are blueprints of the many creations still waiting to emerge. Imagery, like Michelangelo's chisel, cuts through the accumulated layers of fear and destructive beliefs and allows us to lift them out. So each image is a message in a bottle we dispatch into the invisible world. The answer always comes. Our task is to pay attention and learn how to read it. Sometimes the answer comes in a night dream, sometimes in our waking reality. Over the years I've found much solace in this way of working with pictures. What a relief to find that I don't have to rely on my tricky little mind to figure things out. What comfort to lean against an image – an invisible set of hands to take me exactly where I need to be.

Hands of Kindness:

The intention is to allow yourself to feel that you're not alone in your difficulty. See yourself standing in a place of confusion. What are the images, the people, the colors, the smells, and the sounds in this place? Let yourself fully feel and sense whatever comes up. Now feel a pair of kind hands scoop you up and lift you off the ground. Allow yourself to lean against those hands and know in the deepest part of your being that you can trust them to take you where you need to go. Know that you are not alone in your difficulty. As you begin to rise, pictures and clues float into your field of vision, providing you with guidance for the next part of your journey. Let the hands carry you until it's time to descend. Let yourself be gently delivered to a new place of clarity, and peace.

Chapter 6

Mirror of Dreams

"Pay attention to your dreams, they're your
letters from God."

– Jewish proverb

A brilliant young mathematician seeks relief from debilitating headaches. He travels to an island famous for the healing power of its dream rituals. After he is bathed and anointed with oils, he enters a special chamber and drifts off to sleep. A dream comes: He is standing at the foot of a mountain and begins to climb to its summit. As he reaches his destination, he sees a vase filled with liquid. He lifts the vase above his head and turns it over, but instead of water, nine snakes slither down his body, then crawl back up and settle at nine points on his head. Upon awakening, he is healed; his headaches are gone, never to return. The mystery of the number nine revealed in the dream becomes the focus of the young man's work, and he goes on to make his most stunning discoveries.

– Story about Pythagoras

One weekend, my husband Ed and the girls brought home a video of Steven Spielberg's *Close Encounters of the Third Kind.* In the story Roy Neary, played by Richard Dreyfuss, witnesses the arrival of a fleet of flying saucers. Through a language of light and sound the aliens imprint an image deep within him, an image of a mountain, which won't let go of him. His hand draws it on scraps of paper, molds it out of mashed potatoes on his dinner plate. Anguished, Roy pleads for help. "I don't understand what this

is," he says to his wife, "but I know it's important." Ultimately the mountain in Roy's vision turns out to be a repli-
ca of where the first encounter between aliens and humans
is to take place.

Our dreams, like Neary's mountain, are imprints is-
sued from a mysterious Source. They call to us, again and
again, drawing us toward a meeting place where we stand
face-to-face not with an extra-terrestrial but with our own
unadorned self.

I had been actively working with dreams since my early
twenties, but I'd never engaged with them as earnestly as
I did in my quest for a second child. A few months into my
self-healing regimen, a nightmare woke me in the middle of
the night:

> *My ovaries ache and I take a cab to see my gy-*
> *necologist. She tells me I have a cancerous tumor*
> *in my uterus, a punishment for wanting another*
> *baby. Dozens of arms lift me onto a stretcher and*
> *wheel me into the operating room. Several doc-*
> *tors in surgical masks walk in and take turns*
> *bending over me, pressing on my abdomen. "As*
> *soon as you stop trying to get pregnant again,*
> *we'll help you with the tumor," says one.*

Something in me snapped to attention. After eighteen
years of psychoanalysis, I recognized a "child of survivors"
dream when I saw one. Hmm. All those hours on the couch
and part of me still felt undeserving. I'd thought my mind
had closed the Holocaust file long ago, that it was a subject
my various therapists and I had milked for all it was worth.
I understood intellectually, that I was not responsible for
my parents' suffering, or for the engineered slaughter of
millions. But the picture of the surgeons closing in on me

felt like a real, immediate threat. A deep, knowing part of me was asking me to take a good look at it.

I had reached yet another fork in the road. To the left was the familiar road of self-blame, and to the right a path leading to an unknown destination. I attended a prayer service of a wonderful, funny rabbi, Gershon Winkler. A prayer he chanted began: "Dear God, thank you for not letting my destructiveness rejoice over me." My dream might very well have been an answer to such a prayer. Around this time I began experimenting more fully with imagery, and I called upon the pharmacy of my imagination to mix the medicine.

I stand in the middle of a large house with many rooms. Voices coming from behind closed doors question whether or not I deserve to have another baby. I take a silver bell and as I shake it, the doors of all the rooms open and everyone gathers in a circle around me. I face each speaker, respond as truthfully as I'm able to, and choose how much power any of them are to have over me.

Doing the exercise was a little like pouring peroxide on a deep open cut that still sizzled and burned. Stories of my parents' war experiences were emotionally wrenching to think about. But as I allowed myself to remember them, a cleansing of sorts took place. The most painful was the realization that my mother and father had spent a lifetime crippled by unfelt grief. My yet-unborn child showed me an escape route, and let me know I didn't have to follow my parents' fate.

Looking back, my "survivor" dream was a kind of psychic Heimlich maneuver, a shock I needed, to open the airways and clear the blockage that was stopping me not only

from getting pregnant but from moving forward in my life.
Many of my clients think that to really understand
their dreams they must first plow through volumes of
Freud or shop around for a Jungian analyst. In *Fear and
Trembling,* Soren Kierkegaard states: "The truly great is
equally accessible to all." Every single one of us has a direct
connection with the same intelligence that spoke to Joseph
in his prophetic biblical dreams and freed Pythagoras from
his headaches.

"Descend into the dreamworld with the beginner's
mind," I tell my students. "No symbols, no preconceived no-
tions about endowing images with definite meaning." Some
people use tape recorders to prompt them in dream recall.
I'm partial to dream journals. The very first thing I do is
note anything I can summon up. Even if all I'm left with
is a hazy fragment, into the journal it goes. Then I take a
moment or two to close my eyes again, reenter the images,
draw them into the body, and allow them to work through
me. If anything asks to be articulated, even a word or two,
I note it in the journal to jog my memory. This first sleepy
exploration feels a little like driving in heavy fog, but it's
an important part of the process. So turn on your fog lights,
and keep moving ahead until the cottony cloud lifts and you
begin to discern the landscape. An insight seeps in, a tender
place inside you draws the breath a little deeper.

When in doubt, coming up with the right question can
help unravel the most perplexing dream sequence. Of the
following questions, the one that hits the spot in a given
moment is the one I work with.

What is the strongest feeling in the dream? Is there
an image that evokes an intense emotional reaction? Is it a
feeling I'm not ordinarily aware of?

What is the strongest feeling I have after waking up?
Is it different from the feeling in the dream?

How is the dream or any part of it similar to circumstances in my waking reality? Is the dream inviting a new way of seeing those circumstances?

Is the dream validating or rejecting a choice I've made in my waking life?

What direction is the dream moving in? Who am I at the beginning, and who am I at the end of the dream? (Our Knowing Self might be pointing us in a direction of growth, and this question can help us recognize that path.)

If someone I know appears in the dream, why is he/she showing up right now? In what way am I behaving like this person? What is this person's most pronounced character trait? The dream might be letting me know that this trait is a part of me, and I need to become aware of it.

If each dream is an invitation to change something (an attitude, belief, or behavior) in my waking life, what am I being asked to change this time?

These questions are meant to allow images, memories, sensations, and insights to rise up as answers of their own accord. What I find works best is to pose a question, and then if nothing comes just to tuck the dream away and carry it around for a while.

Chances are you will come up with a number of "readings" for a particular dream. But when you hit gold, you'll know it. Dream reading at its best is a kinesthetic experience. The answers we're searching for don't come from figuring things out, but by dropping our questions into the bodymind and waiting, the way one drops seeds into summer soil, then waits. Show a little patience, and soon enough the garden of your intelligence and imagination yields rows of peppers and wild strawberries and flowers of every kind.

Ultimately, you are the only final authority on the meaning of your dream. Your own body and sensibilities are by far the most reliable decoders of the messages you receive. The less cluttered your mind is with theories of symbolism, and the more you open the body to the sensations that rise up, the easier it is to let your own felt physical experience guide you.

Sometimes the Dream Teacher vanishes without leaving a calling card. Not a trace of an image remains. All you know is that somewhere deep inside you all the locks clicked open, and a part of the burden you'd carried had been lifted.

Like any other art, dream reading takes practice. The more attention you give to it, the more rewarding it gets. Then again, sometimes you can have a profound revelation with the very first dream fragment you rescue.

Carol, a forty-something soft-spoken woman with shoulder length, shiny black hair, had one child, a rather persistent one. "Every time she comes home from preschool," she said, talking about her four-year-old daughter, Ruby, "she tells me it's time to go get another baby."

Several months after she joined the Fertile Heart circle in New York, Carol brought in a dream. She e-mailed me a copy a few days prior to our group meeting.

I am making tea for four people in someone else's house. I have to look all over for mugs and tea. Everything is hard to find, not clean. I think if I was in my own house, it would be so easy, I know just where the mugs and tea are, everything is ready. I don't feel frustrated, just persistent, and surprised that the house I am in is such a mess.

As we began to look at it in the group, I asked her to speak the dream aloud from memory. When she did, she left out the part about preparing tea for four people. This was useful for her to notice, because that number was a clear indication that to her inner truth "a family of four" was a possibility. Yet part of her wasn't quite ready to receive this message.

"The strongest feeling I had was surprise," said Carol, "I couldn't believe that the house was such a mess, the mugs were so dirty. But I didn't feel frustrated, just persistent."

As Carol began to speak about the parallels between the dream and her waking life, much shame came up, along with a sense of unworthiness.

"That's the mess I need to clean up before I can be in my own house, before I can have a life and a body that is fully my own. In that house everything would be ready to receive the second baby."

At the following meeting Carol reported that the dream had helped crystallize her unwavering commitment to bring another child into her family. "It's what I want," she told us. "If I don't follow through, I will miss that child for the rest of my life."

Carol's beautiful adopted son Jorge is five months old, and she and several other adoptive moms have helped me organize the first Fertile Heart workshop for people considering adoption.

One way or another, our waking life is an expression of what is inside us, a composite of all the images we've stored. Some of those images we keep carefully concealed from everyone, including ourselves. The good news is that a deep knowing part of us is relentlessly trying to "blow our cover" by giving us a momentary glimpse of that secret reality. "Look," it says, "this is what you're creating, is this okay with you?"

Sometimes, even as we reel in the sharpest silhouette of the secret self, the eye remains too frightened to see it. This is when working with a group or a teacher as witness can make all the difference.

Walking through the door of the Fertile Heart studio in Woodstock in her flowing skirt and green cotton tank top, her auburn hair worn long and free, Andrea exuded the unself-consciousness of someone used to being in the limelight. "My sister's shrink told her that it's my rage that keeps me from getting pregnant. But I don't feel any rage. I'm just sad. I'm really not angry, just so sad," she remarked during the lunch break.

She shrugged her shoulders and looked over at me. "I don't know what to think anymore. It's been three years. I'm tired."

"For now, let's just say that your sister and her therapist might mean well: inviting the raging voices inside us into a conversation can be liberating. But to say that to get pregnant all you have to do is feel your rage is simplistic. Hopefully by the end of the day this will become a little clearer, " I said.

Andrea lived in the suburbs of Philadelphia and worked full-time, so I was surprised when she called to say she would like to join the Fertile Heart open circle in Manhattan. She also said that she'd had a dream that felt disturbing the night after the workshop, and asked if we could work with it in the group.

The following Tuesday evening Andrea brought in her dream:

> *My husband, George, and two of his buddies*
> *are playing baseball in the yard Only they have*
> *no arms or legs; they're pitching and batting with*
> *their heads. In the dream I'm laughing at them,*
> *and tell them they would make a great circus act.*

Her sister's comment about hidden rage must've still been haunting Andrea, because after she finished sharing the dream, she shook her head and said, "I don't see any rage here, do you?"

I was silent for a moment.

"Let's just take a look at one picture frame," I said quietly. "Look at the men again, and freeze that image."

Andrea closed her eyes. A few seconds later she gasped; then her face collapsed and she buried it in her hands and wept. When her anguish quieted, she leaned back against the chair and said:

"My whole marriage is going to hell in a hand basket. George keeps pushing me to do donor egg! He made me go to this depressing talk with two high-powered guys in dark suits!"

She was still weeping, but her voice was growing stronger:

"There's gotta be something better I can do with my time than watch an hour of devastating slides. 'The older you get, the tougher it is' kind of slides. Like it's something I don't know, like it's not stuff that's been shoved down my throat since time immemorial.

"They showed us how – how" she was gasping for breath now, and laughing in relief, "they showed us how the female has the most follicles in utero! That's when we are most goddamn fertile, in our Mother's womb! It's all downhill from there. I bet you anything pretty soon they'll be adding egg retrieval to Planned Parenthood classes. Get those follicles in the fridge while they're still fresh!"

Andrea's cheeks were flushed, but she was calm now, and her face had a new softness in it. "You can't blame me for chopping him up a bit, can you? C'mon, I'm not even forty, I can do this. At least I want to have a fair chance at trying."

Isabel, who'd been part of our circle for several months but so far hadn't done much dream work, was wiping her eyes. "This dream reading stuff really works, doesn't it?" She ventured, looking energized.

"There is definitely something to it," I replied.

Some time later Andrea told me that after that session, she and George went out to a Latin club and danced till dawn, something they hadn't done since their first date. "I told him we had to give up the chase because it's chasing all the fun out of everything we do. I told him I didn't care if it took another five years, I had to do this at my own pace. Whatever it is that's stopping me from getting pregnant, could very well stop me from conceiving even if I use a donor – Oh, yes," she added, laughing a little. "I made him promise no more slide shows."

"And here is the weirdest thing," she continued. "He said he was doing all that stuff because he was scared. He didn't think we could last much longer, the marriage, I mean. He was crying. God, I tell you there is nothing sexier than a weeping man. Do you believe that this was the first time in the eleven years of our marriage that I saw my husband cry? Things with us are better than ever. It's like we're both thawing out."

"We're not pregnant yet," Andrea wrote in a recent e-mail. "But we're having a hell of a good time trying."

A line of Beckett's says it all when it comes to couples caught in the maze of baby making.

"To be buried in lava and not turn a hair, it is then a man shows the stuff he is made of." The consensus seems to be that the stress of fertility treatments and disappointments can easily break up a marriage. Maybe so. But it can also help you find out who you are married to, and what the marriage is made of.

In the all-day Fertile Heart intensive, before we begin our discussion on dream reading, I ask everyone to stand and walk toward the middle of the room. As they walk, I speak.

"As strange or embarrassing as your inner world appears to you at times, there is nothing you can feel or think or imagine that the rest of us wouldn't be able to relate to. Why? Because if each of us were to step into the innermost center of our being, we'd all end up in the same stretch of land, the place where dreams come from, a place where all of us humans speak the same language. Which is why someone's dream in a group will have meaning for everyone present. Each person will find in it the exact medicine she needs."

The moment of anticipation when someone is about to share a dream is one of my favorites. It's as if this person has just returned from an archaeological dig, and she's about to crack open a crateful of exotic objects. The rest of us stand there expectant, marveling at the craftsmanship of each piece, wondering what we're looking at. We hold each object up against the light, amazed.

Here is one of those fine offerings.

The three of us, my husband and I and a little girl, are in a baby carriage. It's one of those old fashioned white wicker ones with a roof. I panic and am about to jump out and start pushing it, but the little girl grabs my arm. She says: No, Mommy, this carriage goes on its own."

When we read dreams as a group, I ask everyone to close their eyes and hear the dream as if it were their own. The images always evoke a particular resonance in all of us.

"As soon as you said my husband and I and our child are in a baby carriage, I saw a bunch of people pushing it. My doctor and my mother, and some other people I didn't recognize. I felt completely at their mercy, had no idea where they were taking us," said a voice, and a number of people nodded in agreement.

75

~~"Our baby was a little boy and he looked older, maybe~~
two. He looked very wise and sweet and patient. It was so
great to be told I didn't have to do anything. It's exactly
what I need to hear today. Also the word old-fashioned felt
good. The old-fashioned baby making had worked for us
once, and I think I want to go back to it for a while." Isabel's
voice sounded patient and wise, as if it carried the echo of
the child in the dream.

Lori, the original dreamer of this lovely fragment, had
a most practical response. Only recently she had suffered
yet another miscarriage. The medical community didn't
offer her, at forty-three, much hope. Lori had resolved to
abandon all medical intervention, to focus on strengthening
her body and heart in every possible way, and to surrender
to whatever was to come next. Her acupuncturist had suggested that in order to heal from the last miscarriage, Lori
and her husband should put baby making on hold for several months.

But this dream had a sense of immediacy and clarity
that said: Go!

"And as you know," she wrote later, "timing is everything."

After five years and six miscarriages, with the help of
her dream Teacher, Lori conceived and delivered a delight-
ful baby boy, who weighed in at a solid 9 pounds, and 20 1/2
inches.

I've said this before, but I for one need to keep hearing
it over and over again. The most useful dream decoding de-
vice by far is the exquisite, innately intelligent machinery
of our own bodies.

"Everything is swinging: heaven, earth, water, fire,
and the secret one slowly growing a body," says the mystical poet Kabir. So is the dream a swing between the reality
of pictures and the verifiable world of tables and chairs.

To enliven the flow of energy between these two worlds, I encourage my students to bring dream elements into the physical world. Why not place the white rose from last night's dream on the dining room table," I ask. "If you keep your eyes wide open, you might notice that the dress you wore in a dream will appear in a store window a few blocks from your office. You can walk in and try it on, or simply breathe in the image and let it land. Another snowflake of hope."

Chapter 7

Issues in Your Tissues

"Kids in distressed families …carry in their bodies
whole arctic wastelands of words not to be
uttered, stories not to be told."

– Mary Karr, *Cherry*

A sorcerer is called to place a curse on a tribe of people. *He mounts his donkey and sets out on his mission, but is soon met by an angel with a sword in his hand. The donkey sees the angel and promptly stops in his tracks. The sorcerer, however, cannot see the angel standing on the path. All he knows is that his donkey is disobedient. And he is not pleased. In his fury he strikes the donkey again and again. Finally, the poor animal has had enough. "You fool!" he calls to his master. "I've been your loyal servant for all these years. If I now refuse to obey, don't you think I must have a reason?" Humbled, the sorcerer sees the angel and realizes that he owes his life to the wisdom of his donkey.*
– Adapted from Numbers 22:1-35

"I was still an honest man," begins a poem of Hungarian poet Ady Endre, recalling a scene from his childhood. A small boy, he stands at the foot of a ladder as his mother climbs to the attic with a basketful of laundry.

> *I was still an honest man.*
> *I stomped my feet and wailed, and begged*
> *Let go of the basket, mother,*
> *and take me in your arms instead...*

We come into the world utterly honest. When we're hungry or hurt, we howl open-mouthed, kick our heels, and flail our arms till someone takes notice. As we grow older we become "well-adjusted," learning to behave and to stay on the adults' good side. The howling and flailing grows a little fainter each day, and we become so good at hiding the truth we no longer even remember it's there.

But the body remembers. It rumbles its grievance through migraines and rashes, cysts and soaring hormones, while we press on, popping a pill here and there to screen out the rising sound.

Then one day, the body, like the sorcerer's donkey, sees danger ahead and refuses to budge.

Part of my evolving self-healing regimen fourteen years ago was a set of yoga postures I did every night. It involved six poses, which I chose according to the phase of my menstrual cycle and my energy level. I usually stayed in each position no more than a couple of minutes. One night I was in the child pose when an image from the birth of my first daughter – a traumatic C-section – floated into my mind's eye. I was being wheeled down a long corridor, with my obstetrician running along the gurney calling to the nursing staff: "Where is the attending? I have to get this baby out NOW!!" The memory brought a wave of panic, and I realized how terrified I was that the next birth would be a repetition of the first.

From that night on, after going through my usual set of poses, I closed my eyes and let the body lead the way. Sometimes my knees folded and began rocking from side to side. At other times I rolled onto my belly, pouring all my frustration into one long stretch. It was the beginning of a meditative movement practice which I later came to call Fertile Heart Body Talk. In a series of movements one can do lying down, standing up, leaning against a wall, or in any number of ways, we give ourselves unconditional permission to physically express and release whatever rises up inside us, as if saying to our bodies: Okay, I see you've been trying to flag me down. Here I am. Talk to me!

Several weeks ago, Rudi, a ten-month-old puppy we adopted from the local pound, taught me a wonderful lesson about body wisdom. It was late at night, and what had begun as a light shower had turned into a summer storm. At the first crack of thunder I heard Rudi whimper and found him trembling in the corner of the living room. I picked him up to calm him, but he kept trembling. We huddled together on the sofa, and he shivered next to me as I dozed off. For the next couple of days, Rudi continued to tremble intermittently. He didn't say, Okay, the storm is gone, I'm safe now, I should stop. His body showed him how to move past the fear and be free again.

Since Rudi's wisdom has been educated out of most of us, chances are we have at one time or another interrupted our knees or our shoulders, or our loyal back, from speaking their piece. Anything we once chose not to experience has been locked away deep within the muscle and marrow. It's like a deposit box you forgot you had because you snuck something in there you don't want to look at. The trouble is, a big chunk of your life force is locked away in that same box.

Given the chance, the first thing the body will ask for is to slow down. Have you ever been late to a meeting? You reach for the last sip of your green juice and trip over the cat, and now the tiles are strewn with glass and the lush white rug is covered with a pattern of green paws. You rip your skirt getting into the taxi and bang your head against the door getting out. That's pretty close to what I imagine the body goes through when we keep pointing at the clock, micromanaging follicle production.

A woman in our community often takes walks with her three-year-old girl. Holding the child's hand, she walks slowly, letting her daughter set the pace. I've seen her carry the child, but I've never seen her pulling her hand or walking ahead. There is something about the tilt of the mother's body that shows complete surrender to the pace of the child. That little girl will grow up trusting her own internal rhythm. Watching them go by, I'm reminded of the small child inside me who knows nothing about rushing for appointments, the child who knows only the wonder of placing one foot in front of the other, and the spaciousness of the present moment.

At first, much of the work is about falling in step with the breath, making a date with our body and permitting it to set the pace without pulling or rushing it, without limiting ourselves to the acceptable or the well- adjusted. Each movement is then the key to one of those forgotten boxes inside of us. We open each one, and unroll ancient parchments that document injustices, crimes, and secrets concealed for generations. We keep to our task, and carefully retrieve everything we find. One of those secret scrolls might hold essential facts omitted from our birth certificate or family scrapbook.

We were meant to slide from the safety of the womb into our mother's welcoming arms. The rest of our lives are profoundly shaped by that first shelter and original meeting. Pregnancy and the birth of a child brings us up close to that memory as nothing else can. Our body knows it. Which is why it sometimes calls: Shields up!

"When I was in your body, Mommy, your feet were my feet, your hands were my hands, your tummy was my tummy. I could eat everything you did, couldn't I?" asked Ariel, the precocious five-year-old daughter of one of my clients, when her mom refused to give her a taste of chili peppers.

"I looked at Ariel and it was like a flash of lightning." Amy told the group one day.

She had been trying to conceive a second child for three years, and since she was now in her early forties, all anyone could say was that she had "age-related-secondary infertility." But now it seemed as though her daughter was offering a second opinion.

"Throughout my entire pregnancy with her I was terrified, and every once in a while this feeling of hopelessness would wash over me. It didn't make any sense. Bill and I were ecstatic about the baby.

"When Ariel said this, I realized that when I was pregnant with her, I was reliving some of my mother's desperation when she was pregnant with me. Desperation I must've sensed when, 'her feet were my feet and her hands were my hands.'

"I thought, yeah, and her heart, her heart was my heart.

"My mother's sister died in a car crash a year before I was born. My mother always said how the pregnancy was a great thing, very healing and joyful. But she must've been still grieving, and scared about all kinds of things. And I went through all that with her. Of course I did!

"What if this second baby isn't coming because I'm scared about having to go through that again?"

Amy shared her revelations with her therapist and continued her Body Truth practice. She sometimes observed herself curling into the fetal position. One day she described her head drawing a figure eight as she lay on her belly pressing her hands against the floor, inching forward, a motion reminiscent of her descent through the birth canal.

Amy's body was doing what it needed to do to feel confident about the next pregnancy. Slowly it began to shed its armor of fear and lead the way. She often reported spontaneously moving through sequences of contractions and release.

Her five-year-old daughter turned out to be her "doctor-teacher" – one with the perfect remedy. And for that she received the perfect reward a year and a half later: a little sister called Naomi.

One day, when I was writing this chapter, a square silver envelope came in the morning mail. I recognized the name of the sender, since Nina had participated in a seminar just a few weeks earlier.

"There is something I have to share with you," said the note. "I've been doing my Body Truth religiously, but afterward I would always feel guilty about giving so much attention to my body. That in itself wasn't that surprising. I usually don't lie down anywhere until I'm ready to collapse, so at first I just wrote it off as a reaction to indulging myself in free time. But I also noticed that I would only do my Body Truth when I was alone in the house. I didn't want my husband to even know I was doing it.

Then a week ago, I was cleaning out some old papers and I found a picture of me and my parents with a man and a woman. At first I didn't recognize them. My mother and I both looked like someone had sucked all the life out of us. Everyone else was smiling. Then I remembered it was a picture from our vacation in Canada when I was twelve. We went to spend a week with a childhood friend of my mother's, whom she hadn't seen in years. They used to be neighbors. He was a real charmer, tall and animated. He asked me a lot of questions and paid attention to me the way my parents never did.

One afternoon my mother and father, and the man's wife went shopping and I was left alone with him. I never told anyone about what happened that afternoon. I think my mother could sense that something was wrong but she never asked about it and I think she was glad I didn't tell her."

Nina went on to write that shortly after the incident she began having debilitating pre menstrual headaches and later developed cysts on her right ovary. She felt that many of her lifelong difficulties, including her struggle to maintain a healthy pregnancy, were in some way linked to the incident. Her Body Truth practice was helping Nina dissolve the dense pit of hurt and anger still inside her.

Two years later, a few days after her forty-fourth birthday, Nina gave birth to a little girl. Attached to the birth announcement was a note: "If you let your body speak, one day it will start to sing." The note continued, "Julia, tell every woman you see to have at least two orgasms before intercourse. They were the snowflakes that finally broke the branch for us."

If you permit it, the body develops its own vocabulary of motion. Approach it with the same tenderness as you would a toddler learning her first words, and little by little it speaks out with more confidence.

"I've always thought of myself as someone who is just not that physical," said Gabrielle, a slim, pensive looking woman with sun-bathed hair, during a recent Fertile Heart weekend workshop.

"But now I'm beginning to wonder about that. Last night I went to my room and I just dropped on the floor exhausted. I didn't have the slightest intention to do anything except to lie there. After a few minutes I found myself scooching into the corner of the room, and rolling onto my belly. I was curled into a tight ball, with my right hand clutching the left. Inside, I kept saying, Leave me alone, just get out and leave me alone! It was like it was all happening without my will. The body was just doing its thing and I was too damn tired to intervene. After a while I went completely limp."

"And I thought," she said, looking around the room, "I don't have to do anything I don't want to. Nothing at all. I mean I've told myself that a thousand times before, but now I knew it through my muscles. This was freedom. Hallelujah!

"It's not that I don't want to have a baby, I do very, very much. But I had no idea that I felt so cornered about it. Like I had to do it for my husband, and my parents, and his parents, and my therapist even. Everybody had a stake in my getting it right. It's the story of my life, doing the right thing for everybody else no matter what it cost me.

"The hell with all that. I'm free! Nobody to please but me. Hey, it rhymes," she said with a smirk. She said it again, this time with the flair of a hard-core rapper, rocking back and forth with her arms folded across her chest: "The hell with all that, I'm free, yeah/nobahdee to please but me!"

"Maybe we can turn it into the Fertile Heart cheer," she said, her eyes lighting up.

Finding your way back into the body, learning what's pleasing and what's drudgery, can do wonders for your sex life. Several years ago, tucked away in the bottom corner of the *New York Times,* was a tiny article about a woman in her sixties who conceived and gave birth to a healthy baby boy. A tabloid ran a photograph of the woman bathing the baby, with her grandchild looking on. It turned out she had a whirlwind affair with her next-door neighbor and her body had remembered something it had known how to do many years earlier.

"I'm not suggesting that you wait till you're sixty," I tell the women in my group, when they begin to talk about timing and position and ovulation kits. "But could anyone argue with the fact that the creation of human life was designed as a supremely pleasurable experience?"

Doesn't it make sense that the most ideal environment for conception is one that makes room for pleasure? When production time is a tedious set of acrobatics, and intimacy and passion are things of the past, sperm get lazy and ovaries get sluggish.

One of the homework assignments I give is meant to stimulate the release of sense memories locked in the tissues. I ask clients to recall an activity they used to love to do in their teens, and to wear colors they liked then, in order to bring back the kinesthetic experience of being eighteen.

Cory, an actress in her early forties, had almost given up hope of a healthy pregnancy after several miscarriages. She took this assignment one step further. "I started wearing my sorority sweatshirt, and all this old stuff about college started coming back. So on a whim, Steve and I decided to drive out to New Hampshire and visit my Alma mater. We walked around campus all afternoon, and you could just smell all those hormones in the air. We stayed in a great bed-and-breakfast, went out to eat, danced, and made love like mad."

And it worked! When Cory's endocrinologist first saw the baby's heartbeat and looked at Cory's promising hormone levels, he told her it was the first time in his twenty-year practice that he had seen anyone with her medical history beat the odds.

One day, my friend Amy and I were leaving a class on biblical text. The focus of the session had been the exodus of the Jewish slaves into freedom. Each day, a cloud had appeared overhead to guide them through the desert toward the promised land.

"Wouldn't it be great," said Amy, "if every morning you got up and there was this cloud floating by, telling you what to do?"

The truth is that our body is an intricate, ingeniously constructed instrument, designed to do exactly what the cloud did for the freed slaves: to show us the way.

Ingrid, at forty-two, was a newlywed. Impeccably dressed, she was always the first to arrive for our twice-monthly meetings, but was wildly resentful of having to make lifestyle changes.

"It took me twenty years to finally meet a man, I'm just starting to have some fun and now you're telling me I can't even go out and get a decent cut of steak? I like French food, and I like wine! "

You would think Ingrid didn't have a whole lot of faith in the work we were doing. Yet though she complained, she didn't quit. In fact, each time she came, she arrived with a larger and larger bag of organic produce from the nearby health food store. One day, I was guiding the group through a Body Truth exercise called the "Wailing Wall." I looked over at Ingrid, who was leaning against the wall, supporting herself with her hands and kicking.

A moment later something inside her gave way, and all the frustration and grief came pouring out in a flood of tears.

Afterward, it was as though Ingrid had entered the Zone. Insight after insight came. She understood how much of her own life was still waiting to be birthed, and that it was not too late for her to be a mother; that it was not too late for her to be the person she'd once imagined she could be. What only weeks earlier had felt like drudgery – yoga, cooking, imagery, and Body Truth practice – had become pleasurable.

The following spring, after a smooth pregnancy and thrilling water birth, I met Ingrid's tiny daughter and her husband at the produce section of the health food store.

We humans listen with delight to sonatas imprinted on sheets of metal and plastic. We sway and swirl to the sequence of notes. As we tune in to the melodic lines of our solar plexus, the cartilage of the knee, and lobe of a lung, the distinction between the useful and the harmful becomes an indisputable physical experience.

Chapter 8

The Ally in the Cupboard

"While I am here, contained within bones and muscles, organs and skin, I want to take care of the gift of my body. I want to feed it well, move it gracefully and rest it deeply."

– Elizabeth Lesser, *Broken Open*

A man and his wife lived in the land of Zorah. The wife was desolate, for she could bear no child. Then an angel appeared before her and said: "Thou shall conceive and bear a son, if thou drink no wine, or strong drink, and eat not any unclean thing." And the man and the woman followed the angel's bidding. The woman bore a son, and called him Samson.

– Adapted from Judges 13:2-5

Food, like imagery, or dreams, or Body Talk, is a tool. A tasty, sweet or sour, crispy or chewy, liquid or solid tool. Another pair of shears to clear the trail. It was through my work with food that I took my first radical step toward self-reliance. For many of my students, *food* is most readily recognized as an agent of change.

"Whatever you do," I tell the women in my workshops, "don't ever go on a fertility diet. Or, worse yet, an *infertility* diet." Though diet books can be useful resources, being on a diet implies a world filled with delicacies that everyone except you can enjoy. Diet is almost always connected in our minds with temptation, deprivation, sacrifice, or even punishment – not quite what you're looking for when you're already feeling excluded and sorry for yourself.

At a recent intensive, Jeff, one of the brave husbands who come to Woodstock dragged by a determined woman, was scanning the handout on food. He and Nancy had been through four years of treatments ranging from drugless intrauterine inseminations to seven in vitros, one of which was a donor egg cycle. Woodstock was the last stop before moving on to adoption. Alarmed by the lengthy "No Foods" column, Jeff remarked, "What do you mean, it's not a diet? Look at all the things we can't eat."

Before he could begin his next sentence, a voice from the other end of the room rang out. I was surprised by the intensity in her voice, since she had hardly uttered a sound all morning:

I think I'm having an aha moment, isn't that what Oprah calls them? " she asked, turning to her husband. "You wouldn't call crossing off sawdust from your menu being on a diet, would you?" Nancy said slowly, holding Jeff's gaze.

"You know those king-size bags of chips we keep restocking every week, the ones we polish off watching the news?" she asked. "I always feel like I'm stuffing myself with salty sawdust. It makes me feel lousy, but I keep doing it anyway."

Sounds of empathy rose from throughout the room and Nancy continued, encouraged by the attentive faces around her.

"I've been torturing myself with food since I was ten. My mother used to stare at my flabby belly every night as I was putting on my pajamas, and she'd shake her head in disgust. I wanted to get rid of those ripples of fat so badly I nearly starved myself to death. I just wanted to get her to stop shaking her head. She never did, never stopped shaking her head. But when I moved out of the house, I started stuffing myself with anything I could get my hands on like there was no tomorrow.

"It just came to me when we were talking about dieting. I know what I've been doing all these years – I've been on an anti-diet. Oh, God!"

As she brought her hand to her mouth, a tired smile lit up her face.

"For thirty years I've been stuffing myself with sawdust waiting for my mother to show up and tell me she was sorry. That I was okay, flab and all."

"You're holding your breath, see if you can allow it to move through you, Nancy. Relax your shoulders a bit," I said softly.

Nancy's voice broke, and tears streamed down her face. "She's been dead for twelve years and I'm still waiting!"

Nancy leaned forward. With one hand she reached for the yellow legal pad containing her notes and held it against her chest. "But you know what? I think I know exactly what to do." She flashed a quick look at her husband, took a pen in her free hand, and drew several quick lines across the page. "I'm crossing – everything – that's in the sawdust category – off my shopping list."

Her husband, a little embarrassed but clearly moved, said with a small laugh: "You're really serious aren't you? And I'm supposed to go cold turkey on this. You realize what you're asking me to do?"

Nancy drew a deep breath and said quietly, "It's your kid asking, not me."

Today, Jeff and Nancy are the blissfully happy parents of two irresistible little girls from China. They made the decision to move forward with their home study soon after the workshop. "Except now we have a pretty good chance to be around for their wedding," wrote Nancy in her last e-mail.

To think of our way of eating as some sort of diet handed down by experts can be wildly confusing. Just about every nutritionist, acupuncturist, homeopath, and medical doctor will give you a different version of the perfect diet. A raw food enthusiast will tell you that eating cooked foods is an addiction, and suggest you join a twelve-step program for cooked-foodaholics; your macrobiotic counselor will caution against eating anything raw, your chiropractor will say absolutely no meat, and your Chinese doctor will tell you to eat lamb. Oh, yes, and none of them will be happy to see you eat white rice and clarified butter, except perhaps that famous Ayurvedic healer who comes to town only once a year and is reputed to have cured everything from repeated miscarriages to the common cold.

So here, once again, if you choose to engage the help of experts, or diet books, allow them to become nothing more than a resource, a voice of support. If to any extent they pull you away from doing your own thinking and consulting your Inner Authority, they're cutting you off from the most reliable guide of all.

Throughout his life, Mahatma Gandhi repeatedly used food adjustments in an effort to heal himself and his family. In his remarkable autobiography, *Experiments in Truth*, Gandhi wrote, "Inhibitions imposed from without rarely succeed, but when they are self-imposed they have a decidedly salutary effect."

When I first came to America, in 1969, after nineteen years in Communist Czechoslovakia, everything I tasted was so much more exotic than anything I had known. I sampled everything and couldn't stop. The clothes I brought with me from the Old Country soon seemed to have shrunk in transit, unless, of course, it had something to do with the twenty-five pounds I put on in the three months following my arrival. At that point I joined the international sorority of calorie counters, and remained a member for the next twenty-two years.

One day, about a year after my diagnosis of "untreatable infertility," I was browsing through a stack of books at the local health food store. A paperback called *Fit for Life* by Harvey and Marilyn Diamond caught my eye. My friend Roberta had mentioned the title a few years earlier, and I had intended to read it ever since. Now I reached for the book, opened it at random, and read: "...*if there's no energy in your body, it means that you're not alive.*" That's it, I thought: of course, energy! Making a baby is no small task. If my body's not doing what I ask, maybe it can't handle the workload. What if, I wondered, I somehow found a way to create more energy?

This simple revelation instantly changed my relationship to food. My meals became the much-needed allies I engaged to champion my cause.

At first, my overall plan was to find a way to increase my energy level. I had no idea how or to what degree this would work, but since no one else was coming up with any "cures" I decided it was worth a try.

It turns out that the body's one most labor-intensive function is...yep, digestion. If we can free up some of that energy, the body will surely apply the surplus to wherever it's most needed: balancing hormones, repairing tissue, perking up cells.

Soon I realized that my body needed mothering before I could move on to parent a second child. This is pretty much true for every woman and man I've worked with over the years. (What's also true is that a large number of these people had digestion-related complaints.)

I began to notice how unconsciously my hand traveled toward my mouth with anything that was even remotely edible; how often I used food as camouflage. Why feel my sorrow if I can drown it in a glass of cappuccino? Why go through the trouble of facing the raging teenager in me when I can silence her with a plate of greasy home fries?

Slowly, I learned to approach my body with the same patient tenderness I'd give to a young child. How do I want to treat her? I asked. How do I protect her from harm, eliminate obstacles in her way, and make her life more pleasurable? Inspecting the aisles of the neighborhood health food store, I picked up a piece of fruit, a jar, and a handful of almonds, and thought: Is this good for my body-child? Is this going to make things easier or more difficult for her? I packed my lunch for the following workday the way I one day hoped to pack my daughter's school lunch. I observed my response to new foods the way a doting first-time mom watches her toddler's reaction to a spoonful of pear mush.

Under the guidance of my ever-so-patient chef-husband Ed, I learned to pick up each ingredient about to go into the mixing bowl and ask: Is this for me or against me? Is this going to make my body hum with joy, or feel as though it's hauling rocks up a steep hill?

The first major adjustment in my way of eating was adapting what much of the holistic literature calls the principles of natural hygiene. There are many ways to go about doing this, but the main idea is simple: Make sure your body has completed yesterday's assignment before you present a new one.

So attend to cleansing and emptying before you offer your digestive tract anything that involves more than minimal labor. Some people might begin the day with miso soup or vegetable broth, others with a glass of hot lemon water, or a shot of wheatgrass. For me, morning cleansing consisted of drinking a tall glass of mixed vegetable juice, sipped slowly so as not to cause an abrupt rise in blood sugar levels. (I'll say more about this later.) After a half hour break I'd have a piece of fruit. Temperate fruits such as apples, blueberries, cherries, or apricots, are best. One of the elements of proper food combining that made supreme sense to me was the idea of eating fruits only on an empty stomach, or as empty a stomach as possible, allowing them to pass through your stomach quickly rather than mix with other foods and cause fermentation or worse havoc.

Since I have what Ayurvedic medicine refers to as Vata constitution, I tend to be cold, so throughout the rest of the morning I'd sip decaffeinated green tea, which I carried around with me in a thermos. On rare occasions when my body asked for more protein, I'd have some soaked almonds or a bowl of grain with miso soup. (This has pretty much been my morning routine for fourteen years, and my stomach has never been calmer.)

Next I began to experiment with the food combining principles articulated in a number of books, including *Fit for Life*. The rule of thumb here was to eat no more than one concentrated food per meal. (Anything that is not a fruit or vegetable is a concentrated food.) I can't say that I always followed this rule, but I did become a lot more mindful of putting together meals that were easier on my stomach.

In my pursuit of an energy-efficient relationship with food I, like Nancy, had to cross off my shopping list items that were depleting my system. Anything that places undue strain on our immune function is not a friend. The vast collection of processed snacks loaded with refined sugar that I absentmindedly munched on throughout the day, the killer fats in prepared salad dressings – these were drugs that were robbing me of minerals and suppressing my immune and brain functions and they might very well have been responsible for some of my chronic ailments and my soaring hormones.

The most urgently needed intervention for me was to learn to sail past the siren song of sugar. When I say that for many of us sugar has been the most difficult addiction to overcome, I'm not citing a survey of the National Institute of Health.

Sweets did not feature prominently on the menu as I

was growing up in Czechoslovakia. But in America, at my uncle's house in Fair Lawn, a New Jersey suburb, dessert was the last course of every lunch or dinner. Soon there was no errand I could go on without picking up a candy bar, croissant, or muffin to keep me company.

Often, somewhere around three in the afternoon, my head would grow heavy and my eyes would glaze over, and I would feel as though I was about to slip into a deep sleep, unless I could quickly wrap my hands around a cup of cappuccino and hold tight till the last drop. This intervention was most effective when accompanied by a slice of cake du jour. And I don't mean the dainty sliver of dessert served in four-star restaurants. I mean one of those hefty helpings of pies lined up in the display cases of New Jersey diners.

It was entirely clear to me that my need for this mid-afternoon snack was a genetic predisposition. Try as I might to curb my cravings, come three o'clock my legs would automatically follow the familiar route. This went on for nineteen years. It was a cyclone of desperation and desire that finally delivered me to a brand-new place. A place where icing and fudge, or even a plate of Hungarian plum dumplings, no longer had power over me.

Thinking back, it was not a question of willpower; after a while those foods simply didn't make sense anymore. Slowly my entire metabolism changed, balance was restored, and cravings stopped.

I found one of the most useful discussions of the "many faces of sugar addiction" in *Mother-Daughter Wisdom*, the book by beloved author, and women's health advocate Dr. Christiane Northrup.

Whether or not a biochemical imbalance is contributing to our sugar craving, if we are to respect the "Onennes of the Human Loaf" we know that the physical body will often mirror the craving of the heart. There is nothing like sugar to cuddle and rock ourselves into oblivion. Only it's not the real thing – it's not the kind of cuddling we're hungry for. Here's an exercise that might be helpful if you'd like to respond to your cravings move creatively:

> *As you're about to head for the freezer or the cookie jar, stop and let the breath move through you. Close your eyes and see the hand reaching for the fix. In your mind's eye see first the hand and then the rest of your body express whatever feelings come up. If you could pour all your feelings into a sound, what would it be? (And if the neighbors are away, go ahead and let it out; if not, a silent scream will work just as well.) Breathe out once. Suppose the hand reaching for the sugar could speak: What would it say? Listen. Let the next breath move through you.*

Now ask yourself: How can I be sweet to myself at this moment? If you still want a cookie, go ahead and have it. Eat it slowly and notice your thoughts and feelings as you do. Sometimes it will take one bite to realize you don't need it anymore.

Wendy usually appeared in group wearing a pair of neatly pressed jeans, a tailored shirt with a white T-shirt under it, and a pair of red cowboy boots. She played the fiddle and made her living teaching music in one of the junior high schools in Manhattan. Several years earlier, Wendy had given up cigarettes and replaced them with candy and cake. I thought the "hand" imagery might offer some clues.

"I get the same image every time," she said at the next meeting. "A starving toddler picking scraps of food off the floor. I don't think this ever happened. We always had plenty of food in the house, but it does feel like I've been living on scraps for God knows how long."

As she continued the exercise, Wendy realized that in spite of her well-stocked cupboards, part of her was perpetually starving. Not for candy bars, or seven-layer cake, but for a sliver of tenderness and attention. A performer and teacher, Wendy was always on the go, giving herself to audiences and students with only scraps of time left over for solitude or for her relationship with her husband, Steve.

With Wendy in mind, I assigned everyone an exercise I learned from John Mann, author of *Divine Androgyny*. The intention of the exercise is to create what I call a Conception Friendly Zone. And again, the idea is to conceive a more intimate, fulfilling relationship, as well as a child. This is what the exercise looks like:

> *Set an alarm clock or stop watch to go off in fifteen minutes. With a partner, place two chairs about twenty feet apart. Sit on the chairs facing one another, silently gazing at each other's face the way one would gaze at a landscape. The idea is to allow whatever comes to rise up, and "to receive" your partner as openheartedly as you can. Thoughts may come and go, but keep going back to your mission: to receive the person before you.*

At the next meeting I asked how the exercise had gone. "I honestly didn't expect Steve to do this with me," Wendy reported. "But all I said was, We have homework to do, and he went, Okay." She looked around at us and giggled. "When we did it the third time, he asked if taking our clothes off would interfere with anything."

A couple of women shrieked with delight. The rest of us cheered.

"Things are getting a lot more interesting in our neck of the woods, let me tell you," added Wendy once the room quieted down.

Judging from Wendy's experience (her daughter Zara was born a week before her forty-fourth birthday) and from reports of couples who included the exercise in their healing practice, the medicinal properties of this low-cost remedy are worth the effort.

So above all, with food as with anything else, cultivate an appetite for truth. What is it you're starving for, and what would be the most constructive way to satisfy your hunger? Do you want rest? Revenge? Attention? Or maybe today it's really just a cookie. The idea is not to judge or to push for change, but rather to be there for yourself as tenderly as you can.

By now it's a pretty widely accepted fact that alcohol and caffeine are not fertility-enhancing foods, by any stretch of the imagination. Like sugar, these foods are akin to addictive drugs. The liver and kidneys, the two main organs responsible for sweeping out the toxins from the body, are also in charge of disposing of any excess estrogen and keeping our hormones in balance. Alcohol and caffeine burden the liver, and eventually our endocrine and our immune system suffer the consequences.

Meat or no meat? is often a question I'm asked. Here again, only you can decide whether or not a vegetarian, flesh-free way of eating is right for you. The minute someone else dictates that decision, a part of you will find a way of sabotaging your efforts. Your ability to choose will grow out of experimenting and carefully observing your body's responses. If you do decide to eat flesh foods, I'd make sure the food is organic, and cruelty and toxin-free. It's also useful to remember that flesh foods are difficult to digest, so you want to give your body plenty of time to work through them. If you choose to eat meat, eat it for lunch rather than dinner. (I'll say more about animal fat and its effect on fertility later in this chapter.)

All this said, most of the women I've worked with have at least lowered their consumption of animal products. Although one client, who later gave birth to a beautiful baby girl, did for a brief period in her healing process eat lamb chops for breakfast several times a week!

The same yes-or-no question often arises in connection with dairy and wheat products. Fifteen years ago, my decision to eliminate dairy was inspired by my chronic sinus headaches. Several sources indicated a strong correlation between milk products and sinus trouble. Amazingly, after three dairy-free weeks, my sinus headaches vanished.

In 1994, the year of my second daughter's birth, a study in the *American Journal of Epidemiology* discussed a correlation between high rates of milk consumption and a decrease in fertility in women twenty years old and older. Digesting the original milk sugar, lactose, produces two smaller sugars, glucose and galactose. The liver then takes up the galactose and converts it to glucose, which enters the bloodstream. Apparently, with some women, this conversion does not happen, and galactose remains and circulates in the blood, causing a number of ovulation irregularities.

Aside from galactose-connected damage, what I know for sure is that dairy products make me feel congested. Many holistic practitioners claim that this kind of congestion can develop in various parts of the body. I've been off diary for many years, but now I do occasionally enjoy spreading a small amount of butter on my toast or vegetables.

Wheat is one of those foods that many of us have difficulty with to one degree or another. Celiac disease, an allergy to wheat products, has been linked to a number of chronic conditions, as well as to fertility difficulties.

So when you first decide to overhaul your eating habits, it's useful to take a three-week hiatus from all flesh foods, diary products, and wheat, and to observe what happens. Then you can gradually either re-introduce these foods into your meal plan or permanently cross them off your list.

Some of my food-related research, such as the subject of proper alkaline acid balance, conjured up memories of high school chemistry. But this time, the stakes were a lot higher than getting an A on my report card. Following is a brief summary of what I came up with on this subject, and why we need to pay attention to it.

Remember the chart of elements you had to memorize in ninth grade? Hydrogen, oxygen, helium...I bet you still remember the little black circle your teacher drew on the blackboard, surrounded by a larger broken circle. That's right, an atom, with the proton in the middle and the electron spinning around it. In most elements, the number of protons is the same as the number of electrons. When the number of electrons differs from the number of protons, we get an atom called an ion. Hydrogen ions are either acid-forming, with needy ions searching for an extra electron, or generous, alkalizing ions with more electrons than they need, looking to donate them.

Just in case you need a brief refresher: When we dip litmus paper into water to measure its PH (potential hydrogen), we're comparing the number of acid-forming ions with the number of alkalizing ions. Watching litmus paper turn from blue to red is another memorable moment. The PH scale runs from 0 to 14, with 0 being the most acidic and 14 most alkaline. The ideal ratio for the human body is between 7.35 and 7.45.

So what does this have to do with food, baby making and energy?

An imbalance between acidity and alkalinity is often

the body's first whimper letting us know that something's off, and alkaline- and acid-forming reactions are an essential part of our personal energy economy. Everything we eat is either acidic or alkalizing, depending on whether the residue left in our bodies after digestion makes us more acidic or more alkaline. (It's not the taste that matters, but the effect. Lemons might be sour, but they have an alkalizing effect.)

Our reproductive organs, as well as all other organs and glands, are constantly seeking to free themselves of excess acids, and our tissues are happiest in an alkaline environment. The more we cooperate in co-creating such an environment, the easier things get. The consensus among clinicians points toward the 80/20 rule, which says that for optimum wellness, 80 percent of our foods need to be alkaline-forming and 20 percent acid- forming. One of the most accessible resources on the subject, complete with lists of foods, is a book titled *Alkalize or Die* by the naturopathic Dr. Theodore Baroody.

Finally, creating energy usually requires some form of fuel. In this case it means a reasonable balance of carbohydrates, fats, and proteins, and all the essential vitamins and minerals. In each of the groups, we'd be wise to learn to distinguish between the good, the bad, and the downright dangerous.

The difference between the good and bad carbs is determined by how quickly they're converted into blood sugar. This is an especially useful distinction when it comes to fertility, since blood sugar levels are directly linked with ovarian function. Foods, such as crackers, bread, chips, and other products made from refined flour, cause a rapid rise in blood sugar. The task of the pancreas is to produce insulin, which clears sugars from the blood so that it can enter into cells and be burned for energy. With frequent spikes of blood sugar followed by production of insulin, some people eventually develop a condition called insulin resistance. One day the cells simply say, *I can't take it anymore!* and refuse to respond to the effect of insulin. This can wreak havoc with our overall metabolism, immune function, blood pressure, and hormone balance, all good reasons to stick with carbohydrate sources such as beans, vegetables, whole grains, and temperate fruits like blueberries, apricots, and cherries.

One of my husband's oft repeated phrases is: Fat is flavor. This is not, however, the only reason you want to include fat on your list of essential nutrients. Fat is also a key player in our endocrine function. Most people do best when roughly 30 percent of their calorie intake comes from fat. But here, too, we should distinguish friends from foes.

The across-the-line bad guys in this group are partially hydrogenated fats, also called transfats, namely margarine, hydrogenated soybean, corn, and cottonseed oil. I'm perpetually horrified to discover how many packaged snack foods (yes, some of them sold in your health food store) are loaded with these anti-nutrients. Transfats are not found in nature. They are manufactured in a manner that renders them a serious health hazard, and their consistent use may disrupt hormones, increase your risk of heart disease and cancer, and contribute to a slew of chronic conditions.

Polyunsaturated fats – such as sunflower, and safflower oil – are chemically unstable, as they react with oxygen; and oxidized fat, promotes inflammation, immune disorders, and cancer, to mention but a few good reasons to keep them out of your kitchen.

An important exception is a class of polyunsaturated fats called omega 3 fatty acids, which are essential for hormone function as well as our overall health. Since our bodies can't manufacture omega-3 fatty acids, we'd be wise to include them in our meal plan. Walnuts, pumpkin seeds, sardines, and herring are good sources of this nutrient.

Saturated fats are mostly of animal origin, and there is much controversy on how much of these fats, if any, we humans can safely tolerate. Those who lobby for radical exclusion of animal fat do so for a number of reasons. The two reasons most relevant to fertility is that animal fats contain both dioxin and arachidonic acid.

Dioxin, an airborne toxic by-product of manufacturing processes which is ingested by animals, has been linked with ovulation irregularities, miscarriages, low sperm count, and poor morphology (abnormally shaped sperm), as well as immune system disorders.

Arachidonic acid induces inflammation of tissues in some people. It turns out I am one of those people, something no one had ever pointed out. So you can imagine how stunned I was when, following my own counsel, I waved good-bye to animal fat, and three weeks later, my lifelong rheumatism and joint pain vanished. If you do decide to include a small amount of saturated fats – like butter – in your food, I'd make sure it's supplied by animals who lived happy lives and were raised on hormone- and antibiotic-free feed.

Finally, the friendly fats are monounsaturated fats, and the friendliest in this group is extra-virgin, organic olive oil. In our family, this is pretty much the only oil we use in food preparation. Ed's approach is to use small amounts of olive oil to stir-fry or saute vegetables. What I do is steam saute with water and add a small amount of oil after cooking.

When I first began experimenting with food, I realized one day that I went pretty much till noon without anything I usually thought of as protein. No eggs, no milk, no buttered rolls. I felt more energetic than I had felt for years but, pouring over volumes of confusing data, I wondered: Am I getting enough protein?

Robert, a naturopath friend of mine, answered my question with a question: "Have you ever met a meat-eating cow or a horse? How do they get enough protein to grow all that muscle ?" he asked. "The amazing thing is that you'd be hard pressed to find a food in nature which doesn't contain some protein. "Every vegetable, or fruit, every ounce of wheatgrass juice you sip, has protein in it. Most people in our culture have to worry not about getting enough, but getting too much protein."

By no means do I wish to underestimate the importance of protein as a nutrient, especially since it's essential for building new tissue. Certainly, when preparing for pregnancy you want to eat a variety of protein-rich foods. Nuts and seeds, beans combined with high-protein grains such as millet and quinoa, and a small amount of animal protein (sardines, herring) for those who are not strict vegetarians are great options.

My conversations with holistically minded physicians and nutritionists confirmed Robert's concern about the hazards of eating too much protein. Protein molecules are more complex than fat or carb molecules and much more difficult to break down, so as an energy source, protein is not the fuel of choice. And that's not the only thing. Protein molecules contain nitrogen, and after digestion they leave a residue of amino acid waste. The liver and kidneys are then called on to cleanse the body of the flood of this amino acid ash, and sometimes their cry for help takes the form of autoimmune disorders, allergies, estrogen dominance (the liver is the organ responsible for elimination of extra estrogen), and other symptoms. The consensus at the moment is that roughly twenty percent of our diet should be protein.

A number of useful resources have discussed the role

of vitamins and minerals in our overall wellness, and of course our fertility. Ours is a culture that loves the promise of the quick and easy, the salvation of pills and magic potions, and remedies that will do the job without any effort on our part. A subliminal message behind the advertising of many supplements is that if we find the right brand we won't have to worry much about the food we eat or the life we lead. So let me haul out my sign again: The genie in a vitamin bottle might seduce and dazzle and even produce temporary results, but anything we don't attend to with care and patience and persistence will eventually catch up with us. Having said that, I do find that some supplementation with vitamins and minerals can be useful, as long as we remember that the most reliable source of these nutrients are foods that are as close to the way they're found in nature as possible. No man- or woman-made supplements can compete with the genius that blends the mix of antioxidants in a blueberry or the brand of calcium in a leaf of kale.

Medicinal plants are a form of food, so here is some input on herbs. Much controversy and confusion arises around the safety of herbal remedies. Some time ago I attended a lecture by a fertility educator who raised little concern about the possible side effects of pharmaceuticals, but spent considerable time expounding on the dangers of common Western herbs. Her argument was based on a study that showed the popular herbal remedies Saint John's wort, ginkgo biloba, and echinacea to potentially interfere with the reproductive process. St. Johns Wort, gingko biloba, and echinacea are not fertility-enhancing plants, and it's useful to know that they are counter indicated for reproductive health, but that doesn't in any way diminish the medicinal value of plants. (It stands to reason that you wouldn't take herbs if you're taking hormone stimulants.)

Near the stream behind our house are lovely patches

of nettle, a blood builder and a popular fertility tonic. Harvesting it and making an infusion is one of the great joys of country living. If you are drawn to herbal remedies, I suggest you turn for advice to women and men who have spent a lifetime studying them. Herbs are useful because of their medicinal properties, so you want to know what those properties are before you ingest them, and you want to carefully observe your body's response. As with any other medicine, the idea is to give the internal healing system a boost, and to remove impediments that keep it from functioning at optimum levels. With that in mind, I would not use hormone stimulating herbs for extended periods of time.

Nutrition is a relatively young science: What's dogma today is highly controversial tomorrow, and dismissed six moths later. Much of what I've discussed here are simple, common sense principles you can verify or disprove through your own experimentation. It's a project that might not only increase your chances of conceiving, but give you what it takes to chase your little one up the monkey bars.

In one of the last scenes of *Annie Hall*, Woody Allen turns to Diane Keaton and says,

"A relationship is like a shark. It has to constantly move forward or it dies. And I think what we have on our hands is a dead shark."

Our relationship with food also needs to keep moving forward. The most important principle of healthy eating is the Pleasure Principle. You know that something's working when you begin to have fun doing it. (This, by the way, is true not only with food, but with everything else in your healing practice.) My hope is that you engage in this exploration not through the power of your will, but through the power of your imagination and an appetite for adventure. There is always more fun to be had: finding a new way to saute asparagus, seeing if you can reproduce the foamy pink raspberry soufflé your mother made on Sunday afternoons; rising to the challenge of a spring fast, or getting some seeds and planting daikon on your balcony. Without such adventures, what you might end up with is a dead drag of a diet.

One last thing: Remember that you are a one-of-a-kind creation. You don't have to do this the way your friend did, or the way I did it, or the way your diet book says it's done. Diet books, articles, and research studies are terrific resources; they're learning tools that provide information, inspiration, and even recipes. But only your body can tell you what it wants for breakfast tomorrow morning. And only by giving it your undivided attention can you find out whether your choices energize or deplete you.

For me, choosing to eat well is an extraordinary way to participate in the food chain and to show my solidarity with every living thing: the blue jay perching on the bird feeder near my window, the soil that has brought forth the red pepper on my plate, the spring air drawn into my daughter's lungs as she pumps her legs and leans against the back of the swing. The stuff I place in my shopping cart at the market will either nourish or harm me and the things I cherish. Making life-affirming choices makes me part of a much bigger circle, and if I listen closely I can hear the blue jay and the pepper and the breeze rooting for me.

Choosing to eat well is also the most fitting way I know to be grateful for my life, and perhaps, that is the best possible reason for deepening our relationship to food. No matter what our circumstances, some part of us knows a *thank you* is in order. When all our other truths have been said and done, the only appropriate thing we humans can say is this: Thank you.

Part Three

Truths and Consequences

Chapter 9

The Seventy-Six Orphans
and the Ultimate Mom

"Every woman who heals herself helps heal
all the women who came before her, and all
those who come after her."

– Christiane Northrup, M.D.
Mother-Daughter Wisdom

*M*ilarepa was a fearless sage who could face just about any situation without blinking an eye. During the day he appeared whenever he was summoned and performed acts of unmatched bravery. Everyone was in awe of his courage.

But each evening when Milarepa returned to his simple hut after a hard day's work, a dragon would be waiting for him: monstrous, fire-breathing, foul-smelling. The terrified Milarepa tried flattery, bribery, and threats, everything he could think of, to get rid of the dragon. Nothing worked.

One evening, desperate and worn out, Milarepa couldn't take any more. With his eyes shut tight and his fists clenched in terror, he called out: "Open up those jaws as wide as you can, I'm coming in!" In that moment, the dragon disappeared.

– Tibetan legend

The longing to create life springs from the deepest, most tender place within us. But it is also the place where we have stored away every sorrow too frightening to face. It is what makes this challenge so painful, and it is also what makes it a most extraordinary opportunity. In a scene from the movie *Defending Your Life*, Meryl Streep shows what she's made of when, without the slightest hesitation, she runs back into a burning house to save her cat. For most of us, life at one time or another feels like a burning house, with walls collapsing all around. The only thing we can do is run for it, while parts of us remain trapped under the rubble. Much of the ache of the baby search comes from those abandoned pieces of ourselves.

Now that we are older and stronger, the good news is that we can go back in and begin our rescue mission. Amazingly, each time we walk through the flames, and dig through the next heap of debris, another part of us springs back to life. Little by little we begin to put ourselves back together, and our hearts and minds and bodies start to unclench. Everything, including conception, becomes a whole lot easier.

For me, the diagnosis of "irreversible, hopeless infertility" meant I was different from all the other mothers around me, for whom a second pregnancy seemed as effortless and perfectly timed as the first. This brought back part of me that had always felt irreversibly, hopelessly different from others. It brought back a young girl ashamed of her home, her Jewishness, her loneliness. A girl who was confused by such feelings, and utterly powerless to change her circumstances.

But this was also a chance for that young girl to speak and be heard. I dreamed up the Garden of Truth imagery exercise to enable this to happen. It's an exercise I often use to work with difficult feelings.

See and sense yourself standing in front of a silver gate. The gate has a plaque with your name inscribed on it. It is a gate leading into your Garden of Truth. Open the gate and step inside. Breathe out once. Allow yourself to fully experience all that you are feeling at this moment. Now look directly in front of you and see a gazebo made entirely of glass. You are able to see everything that happens inside. In the gazebo is a child who feels exactly the way you are feeling at this moment. Notice this child's clothes, including their colors and any objects that might be around. Let this child express all that she needs to express as fully as possible, through her voice, her body, and any sounds she wishes to make. Allow any other people who should be part of this scene to enter. See if there is anything that needs to be said, or done. Breathe out once. Now step inside the gazebo, and if there is anything you wish to do or say to anyone, do so as fully as you can. If you'd like to talk to the child in the gazebo, or comfort her, do so in any way that feels appropriate. Whenever you're ready, say good-bye, and leave the Garden of Truth the same way you entered it. Know that you can return there anytime you wish.

Breathe out and open your eyes.

Laura, a twenty-nine-year-old woman whose menstrual cycles stopped after her mother's death, said during a Fertile Heart phone circle: "I can't take all this pain. I go to the movies, I go for walks, I try to do all kinds of things, but it keeps following me wherever I go. I can't shake it."

I spent so much of my life turning away from the truth that I can certainly appreciate the temptation to run from pain. At the same time, it's become quite clear to me that pain, rage, loneliness, and grief are the fire-breathing dragons that live in every human heart. Sooner of later the only thing left to do is walk right up to them and say, "Open up,

I'm coming in." As soon as we do that we find that inside their dragon suits are abandoned, gentle creatures, little baby dragons hoping for someone to hold them close and shield them from harm.

In the language of the Fertile Heart Practice, we call these dragons the Seventy-Six Orphans. There is also an unconditionally loving, patient, and wise voice within us which I have come to call the Ultimate Mom. Her job is to attend to those abandoned Inner Orphans. Sometimes all you need is one person who will see how generous, brave and breathtakingly lovely you are. And many of us have to first find that person inside ourselves.

Cultivating the presence of the Ultimate Mom is about learning to be militantly on our own side, asking ourselves over and over again: Is this useful? Is this the kindest course of action?

Once we begin to observe our behavior through the eyes of the Ultimate Mom, telling the truth becomes a lot less threatening.

For years I have ached for a cozy, ordered home, the kind I imagined everyone but me had, while growing up. We have now been living in Woodstock for three years, and there are plants on the windowsill, a green sofa against the wall, and cotton beige curtains draped on each of the windows. But the long empty living room is comfortless. My heart yearns for solace and beauty, but my interior decorators are hired by the orphans in me. Right now I'm just not ready to hear their stories. If I did they would remind me of the cold, cracked stone floor in the kitchen of my childhood. They would speak about coming home alone after school in the dark, late winter afternoons, and walking to the far end of the yard to the shed. No doubt the orphans would remind me how scared I was as I opened the rickety door, reached in for the shovel, and trudged with a coal-filled bucket back to the house.

I'd remember how glad I was when the house was finally warm, and in my mind's eye I'd see my mother walk through the door.

I would have to remember all that, and I'm not ready to. Not yet.

It's not like I'm giving up on the dream of a comfortable home. It's just that for now I must tell the truth: My fear of these stories is stronger than my desire for a lovely living room.

"How does the rose ever open its heart and give to the world all its beauty? It feels the encouragement of light against its being, otherwise we all remain too frightened." says the mystical poet Hafiz. What if a difficulty, or an unmet desire, is a hand pressing against the small of your back that says: "Keep going!"

I tell my clients that when something hits a nerve, when the pregnant woman on the bus makes you feel as though there is only one more baby to be had, and she's got it – if you just stay with that feeling for a while, you may find something out. Maybe you grew up with a father who came home drunk every night; maybe you always felt that by the time it was your turn to get a dad, all the good ones were gone. And your inner Ultimate Mom may need to sit and be with that cheated part of you, so that you don't spend the rest of your life living out that story.

The father of one of my clients was murdered when she was twelve. (I talked about her briefly earlier in the book.) Etched into the graceful lines of Ellen's features was a kind of numbness, an expression of chronic grief. When she first shared the story of her dad's murder with the group, we sat in stunned silence for a long time. In the months that followed, Ellen worked on a number of imagery exercises that amplified the voice of the Ultimate Mom within her and

~~brought back to life~~ parts of her that had been numbed by unfelt pain.

"Our family never talked about my dad's death," she said, her face softened by sorrow. "We all grieved in our own way, but my mom felt so overwhelmed herself she didn't know how to help me."

Now, Ellen was learning to help herself. Later, she decided to move on to adoption while continuing to work in the group, as well as with a private therapist. But she found a way to turn grief into a life force rather than pass it on to her future child.

This task of soothing the orphans, of smoothing out ancient scars, is never done.

Some of those Seventy-Six Orphans inside us often prefer to stay in hiding. Being rescued would mean surrendering to the unbearable reality that the original culprit will not be returning to set things right.

No matter how many times she resolved to arrive on time, after three months of being part of the group, Chris, a red-haired managing director of a large marketing firm, consistently walked through the door just a few minutes after we began. As she distractedly surveyed the room, then slipped the jacket of her dark tailored suit quietly off her arm, it seemed as though part of Chris was still reviewing the fine points of a marketing campaign. By the time she fully "arrived," a good chunk of group time was gone. Others occasionally came late; Chris was tardy every single time. It was upsetting for her and becoming disruptive for the rest of us.

I decided to try an experiment, not only to offer Chris a chance to become more aware of what was troubling her, but also to deepen the work in the circle.

"We're only meeting once every two weeks and our time together is precious," I said one day. "I know how tough it is for all of you to navigate traffic and office meetings and clients and make it here on time, but let's make a commitment as a group to do it anyway. At least let's try, shall we? Next week the doors will close at six o'clock sharp and we'll go on with the circle as is. If there are only two people here, well then, it will be a very small group.

"I'd like to try this for two months and see what happens. Afterward we can decide to keep this arrangement or go back to the way things are now."

The suggestion was greeted with enthusiasm.

On her way out Chris flashed me a defiant look that said: I'll be here; count me in.

But at the next circle, two women were missing. Chris was one of them. For a minute I began to second-guess my efforts to raise the bar, but the work was so much more focused that evening that I decided it was a good decision after all.

Still, I was sad to have possibly lost Chris.

Two weeks later, as I walked in at a quarter to six, a woman in a beige dress and blue silken scarf was brushing her hair in the far corner of the room. That must be Jennifer, who e-mailed me to say she'd be attending today, I thought, but as I walked over to introduce myself, the woman turned gracefully, and there stood Chris.

Laughing at my expression, she said triumphantly: "I swear, I feel like I broke out of jail. At five o'clock I closed the door to my office, took off my suit, put on a dress, and waltzed out of there with everyone gaping as if I were stark naked. You don't understand: This is huge! Nobody leaves at five, nobody, it's just not done."

Chris took out a silver clasp and pulled back her hair.

"I was actually early enough to get a snack and walk part of the way," she added, as both of us found our places in the circle and settled in.

A couple of sessions later, Chris said she was having trouble with an imagery exercise I'd assigned, and I suggested we do it as a group.

"Please sit up, straighten your spine, close your eyes, and let the breath move through you," I began.

"See yourself standing at the doorway to your heart," I said. "Know that the Ultimate Mom is waiting for you behind the door. Knock. Watch the door open. You are greeted as you always knew you would be. Welcome home!

"Breathe out, a long, slow out breath, and open your eyes."

The faces around the circle looked softer, less guarded. Chris spoke first: "When I did it on my own it was my mother who was waiting behind the door, and she was a mess. *I* was the one who had to take care of *her*.

"But this time it was way different. I opened the door and this ten-foot-tall woman, all in white, came toward me and just scooped me up and held me. I was very small and weak and it was okay...it was okay for me to feel weak.

"I'm so sick of keeping it together for everybody else, first my mother and, now that she's gone, my sister. She's not a happy person, and I don't think she's ever going to be with anybody. And then sometimes she is as sweet as can be and I open up to her, and make a simple request. I tell her to stop reporting to me about every miscarriage in the neighborhood and *bam!* I get into a direct line of fire.

"Now she keeps asking me about the next IVF, but I know she doesn't want me to have a kid. Who's gonna take care of *her?*"

Listening to Chris, I thought about how so many of us choose to suffer out of loyalty to the suffering we grew up with, and to the people we love, who may have lived and died imprisoned by their circumstances.

"The way to help your sister," I said to Chris, "is to live

the best life you can. To show her what's possible."

The group went on to talk more about choosing to be fully alive as the only way to inspire change in someone else. In choosing to be fully alive, we even have a shot at changing the past. We can redeem the lives of those who came before us, the lives of our mothers and grandmothers, however flawed or traumatic they may have been. They become part of the current that brings forth our own creations, be they children, works of art, or anything else we contribute to the world.

A woman sitting next to Chris turned toward me and said, "My sibling situation is a little different." Jackie's voice was thick with a sense of urgency, as if she wanted to get the story out as quickly as she could and be done with it.

"My sister got married six months ago, and every time the phone rings I think it's her calling to tell me the *great news*. It would be just like her, all she ever had to do is flash a smile and everybody would be eating out of her hands. My parents were always falling all over themselves, ready to shine her shoes or wipe her nose. I'll bet you anything she'll have *twins* by Christmas. By now Jackie was laughing hysterically, though I was not at all sure that she wasn't about to cry.

"I know that's sick," Jackie said finally gathering composure. "I keep telling myself I'm not a bad person. I love my sister, of course I want her to have kids, but if she gets pregnant anytime soon, it'll kill me."

"I don't think it's what you want to hear, but I'll say it anyway," I said to Jackie. "Maybe right now your sister is your greatest healer. Her pregnancy might coax one of the orphans crouching in some corner out of hiding, Maybe that orphan is a little girl who has been trying to get someone's attention for years."

Several weeks later Jackie had another, her third, miscarriage, and this time she gave that young girl inside her full permission to rage and grieve in a way she had never done before.

"I've been thinking," she said slowly at our next meeting, tucking strands of hair behind her ear, "that maybe right now, bringing that orphan out of hiding is more important than getting pregnant?"

"Maybe so," I said as gently as I could.

"That's hard," she replied, her lips trembling.

"I know."

Jackie started to trust her instincts more and more as she dove deeper into the work. Earlier, she had been tested for the presence of anti-phospholipide antibodies – a condition that causes blood clots and cuts off the flow of nutrients to the baby – and was told this was not her problem. Now, reading the stories of women diagnosed with this condition, she intuitively felt this was exactly what she was up against. Jackie insisted on being retested. This time the test came back positive.

During her next pregnancy she was injected with a blood-thinning agent for the entire nine months. Zach, her little boy, was born on December 22, just in time for Christmas.

The mind, says a familiar adage, is like a parachute: It only works if it's open. The heart, too, can only do its job if it remains open. And goes on perpetually opening wider and wider. Only then can it continue with its discoveries. There are countless stories I've witnessed that have showed me the astounding power of the heart to sabotage or aid our efforts. But there is one, or should I say four, that I particularly love to tell.

In a two-year period shortly after I began teaching the Fertile Heart work, four women in different parts of the country came to hear me speak. They had been trying to conceive for up to five years, and had gone (except for one) through several stimulated cycles as well as months of acupuncture and diet changes. The diagnoses varied. One had soaring follicle-stimulating hormone levels and acute menopausal symptoms, one had stage three endometriosis, and two suffered from repeated miscarriages. By the time they came to hear me speak, all of them had been given a very poor prognosis and were advised to consider donor eggs or adoption as their only chance of parenting.

The four women had one thing in common: Each was adopted soon after birth.

When we first talked after the workshop, I applauded their lifestyle changes and their persistence. I also said that regardless of the diagnosis, at the center of the difficulty for each of them was the fact that they had not fully healed the deep hurts connected with their own coming into the world.

"It's something I thought about for years," said Sonya, a spunky sociologist, when I first suggested that her history was where I'd begin to search for clues.

"I have so many unanswered questions about how exactly things happened and why I was given up for adoption and who my birth mother was, but I was afraid to hurt my mom and dad. So it was never really discussed, not really."

Within two months, Sonya found, contacted, and met her birth mother and birth father, and discovered the most astonishing details about who she was and why the adoption had happened. Sonya also participated in the support circle and worked diligently with specific imagery and movement sequences. Slowly she began to view her past and everyone in it with deepening compassion.

Sonya and the other three women had come to understand the many confused beliefs and fears connected to motherhood and birth.

Naomi wrote me a card sharing some of her revelations: "My mom told me so many stories about the years of trying and disappointments and finally how grateful and thrilled she and dad were when I showed up. If I get pregnant, I'll be betraying her. I'll be aligning myself with my birth mother, someone who had abandoned me. I know that sounds pretty twisted but I really think it's what I had felt for years.. "

Within five months of beginning their inner pilgrimages, all four women conceived and then went on to give birth to beautiful healthy children. Two of them have publicly shared their stories.

Adoption is a miraculous parenting option. When we go through it with wide open eyes, it can help us heal a lifetime of wounds. Many spiritual traditions teach that the adopted child is a source of extraordinary blessings, since it brings healing to two family lines. But, as many adoptive parents tell me, adoption doesn't instantly erase years of disappointment and loss. Nor does it dissolve all our ambivalence in a day. With the adoptive process as with anything else, everything we turn away from – our sense of failure; the feeling of being cheated, or unworthy – might one day find expression in our children's emotional lives.

In Mitch Albom's poignant novel *The Five People You Meet in Heaven*, heaven is the place where you get to understand what your life was all about. The sacred links that connected one event to another, the people who showed up just at the right time to provide the next guidepost, are revealed in a beautifully crafted story.

Knowing that your life has meaning feels like heaven. But you don't have to die to get to a place where you begin to discover that you have arrived here as an envoy of Truth; that your most urgent task is to clear up the debris of delusions accumulated in the corner of the family estate, and to restore balance on the acres of land you've been assigned to tend. Even if your child were to appear tomorrow, you shall not find true rest until you set out to get that job done.

Ellena, my older daughter, is at a language immersion camp in Minnesota. *"I'm so homesick, two weeks seems like forever. Don't do anything exciting without me. I love you to the fullest, Mommy,"* she writes on lined yellow notepaper. Two weeks later she's back, belting out an endless string of Italian songs, her eyes lit up, her laughter spilling through the house. My entire body tingles with happiness for her. I think of my mother standing at the turnstile in Vienna as I boarded the plane for America. It was meant to be a summer vacation, but remembering her smile as she waved good-bye, I realize she must've known that I was not coming back. I think of the pain that must have caused her. Feelings well up in me. Missing my mother, praying for my daughters to find their way. It hurts to feel so much. Let it come, whispers a voice in my head; let love come and I promise to use it well.

Strengthening the Ultimate Mom instinct means learning to trust that which is difficult. The stronger the heart, the more we allow ourselves to remember, to see, and to understand. How else but through our own pain are we to learn about compassion? How else will we be able to stand by and allow our child to feel whatever grief he or she may need to feel in order to grow and become fully human? How else will we hear the cry of the children born into entrenched poverty and violence – children suffering the consequences of disease epidemics, famine, and war in countless places around the world – unless we embrace the unending caravan of orphans within ourselves?

Chapter 10

Celestial Gravity

"Swift wind! Space! My Soul!
Now I know it is true what I guessed at;"

– Walt Whitman, *Leaves of Grass*

A small child found an egg, and, not knowing what kind it was, placed it alongside all the other eggs in the warm nest of a mother hen. A little while later the eggs hatched, and lo and behold, among the chicks an eaglet appeared. Since the eaglet knew nothing about eagle ways, she grew up pecking and clucking around the yard just like all the other chickens. Then one day she heard the call of an eagle and looked up at the sky, amazed.

She turned to Mother Hen and asked, "Who is that?"

"Oh, that's the great eagle, the queen of all birds," replied the hen. "She circles the sky; we chickens circle the ground below."

"Come!" the eagle above called out one last time. But the eaglet had already returned to clucking and pecking. She remained a chicken till the end of her days, and never learned that she, too, belonged to the sky.

– Russian folktale

Adi, at eleven, is now the one who reads out loud to me during our nightly ritual. Not long ago, we read Sharon Creech's magnificent novel *Replay*. In one of the chapters, Leo, the protagonist in the story, tells how his father bends over his reluctant rosebushes each summer, coaxing them into bloom.

As I drifted off to sleep later that night, I thought that we humans are like the rosebuds in Leo's garden. And I thought of God as a gardener, bending over us, gently touching the stem of our lives, pruning, watering the droopy leaves, patiently coaxing us into bloom.

It seems odd to acknowledge this now, but in spite of years of mystically inclined workshops, a brief foray into Buddhism, and a myriad of meditation practices, words like *spirituality*, *grace* or *faith* carried no meaning for me. They were not linked with any particular feeling or experience. Much of my life I knew that something in me was starving, but I would not have been able to name what it was I hungered for, or where I ought to look for nourishment.

The Hungarian prayer my mother taught me when I was a child remained the only prayer I knew for much of my adult life.

> *Dear God, sweet God*
> *My eyes are closing*
> *But yours remain open*
> *Please watch over me as I sleep*
> *Watch over my mother and father*
> *And over my dear sister*
> *So that when the sun comes up tomorrow*
> *We can embrace one another once more.*

As I would whisper the words into my pillow, part of me was certain that they ascended to the heavenly realm, successfully enlisting protection. But it was not a part of me that either my parents or my teachers or any adults around me acknowledged. Communist ideology saw religion as the opium of the masses, designed to keep oppressed people in bondage. Though religious practice was not officially banned, it was best not to be seen anywhere near a church or a synagogue, if you hoped one day to send your children to a university, or wished to ever have a decent job. My mother had a deep love for the spiritual teachings of her tradition, and an equally deep ambivalence about how much of that love was wise to pass on to my sister and me. On High Holidays, she sat bent over the pages of her prayer book, yet I never heard her utter a Hebrew word out loud.

My younger daughter's arrival is an event I will celebrate all the days of my life. And the pilgrimage that led me to Adi brought another astonishing gift. From that first pivot of awareness which compelled me to change my eating habits, I sensed that something extraordinary was happening to me. It was not until years later, when I shared my experience with others, that I began to understand the magnitude of this gift. Mirrored in the faces of the women who sought me out, I saw a familiar desperation. A desperation that came from a hunger deeper even than the hunger for a child. The journey we were on was a soul-driven quest to acknowledge, experience and celebrate the spiritual side of our own nature, and of all of creation.

A perfect mix of longing and stored sorrow became the exact force we needed to finally pull us across the border to freedom. To the land we had been searching for all our lives. To a land in which the Wisdom that guides us is a palpable presence. There are as many ways to reach this land as there are people. You don't need a passport or a visa; you don't need anyone's consent to begin the journey, or a permit to operate an approved mode of transport. All you need is a willingness to board whatever vehicle presents itself. Sometimes it looks like a devastating lab report, sometimes a pumpkin with a quartet of gray rodents. If you're willing to trust the vehicle, it can get you to the ball.

The emotional and the spiritual realms are often

treated as two distinct subjects. I have assigned separate chapters to each of them in this book, but it is hardly possible to speak of one without the other. The clearest view of the landscape of the Soul is from the summit of the Heart, where we are still unaffiliated, loyal to no other master but our own truth. And there is no more trustworthy sherpa to help negotiate our ascent than the *Mother, Lover, Sister, Dreamer, Defender of Justice* – the *Fertile Female* within each of us.

"Look at me," she says: this is who *you* are too!

At times I envision her standing tall, rooted in the earth, an infinite number of slender strands streaming from her fingertips, carrying sustenance to all of creation. Once in a while she tugs at one of the strands to pull us out of harm's way. Compelled to pass on my story as clearly as I can, I scrub away layer after layer of borrowed truths, and the constricted vessels inside me open to receive her nourishment. I feel her voice rising, speaking through me, validating my own knowing feminine self.

Revered by millions of people across the centuries, the Fertile Female enables each culture to draw strength from their own vision of her. She is Kwan Yin, the Buddhist goddess of love and compassion, or the tall Yei Be Chai corn goddess in Navajo weaving. My friend Brigitte named her daughter, Cerridwen, after the celtic goddess of wisdom. Sue Monk Kidd's wondrous novel, *The Secret Life of Bees* is centered on the fierce, protective authority of the Black Madonna and a young girl's coming of age. Earlier this year, a reader from Australia sent me a woman's prayer from the Aboriginal tradition that begins:

Great Spirit, I am Mother.
I was made by You
So that the image of Your love

Could be brought into existence
May I always carry with me
The sacredness of this honour.

In mystical Judaism, Shekinah is the earth-dwelling resplendent bride of the Creator. One of my favorite moments in the Friday night prayer service, which marks the beginning of the Sabbath, comes when a member of the congregation walks up to the door, opens it wide, and the rest of us bow as the invisible Shekinah steps across the threshold of the sanctuary

During a recent workshop, Larry, a stoic man in his early fifties, was suddenly shaken by sobs.

"I had no idea, no idea," he sighed as he and his wife said good-bye at the end of the day. "I thought I was just coming to be here for Kate. I thought I was doing just fine. The only other time I remember crying like this was when my dog got run over by a car. That was forty years ago... I have a lot of catching up to do."

Men need to evoke the presence of the feminine even more urgently than do women. Just as there is both a feminine and masculine aspect of the divine, so are they both intrinsic attributes within each of us. When we deny one or the other, we deny an essential piece of ourselves.

My neighbor Margaret, a real estate agent, tells me that in real estate it's all about "location, location, location." In the realm of the Soul, it's all about attitude, attitude, attitude. Spirituality, as I see it, implies an attitude of Faith: to allow for the possibility that wherever we find ourselves at any given point in our life is the best place for us to be. Someone recently posted a note on the Fertile Heart message board: "I hadn't had a menstrual cycle in sixty-three-days but it's back, two days after the workshop I started bleeding. It's a miracle: God is good."

The miracles that bring what we've been wishing for are easy to celebrate. But what if a sixty-three-day stretch without a menstrual cycle, or a diagnosis, as frightening as it is, is also miraculous?

As sages have proclaimed for thousands of years, nothing in creation is not a miracle. Attempting to adapt this view does not preclude groaning, and grieving, or feeling shortchanged and excluded – as long as somewhere inside us a door remains slightly ajar. As long as we remember that we may not have all the answers. Perhaps each of our difficulties is the call of our truest self trying to tell us we're eagles trapped in our earthbound chicken habits; a reminder of the life we had once intended to live. This small shift in our perspective allows us to view a challenge as an unfolding of a mystery, rather than an affliction we must cope with and overcome.

I do admit that looking at crisis this way is a radical proposition. It runs so contrary to the way most of us have been conditioned to approach life that I for one have to remind myself of it each time God appears to have misplaced my latest wish list. But over the fifteen years since my diagnosis I've been – very, very slowly – learning to "bow to what is." That does not mean that I passively wait for a rescue team. Faith is the river I drink from when I've been drained dry. Then I refill my water flask and hit the trail again. Even as I surrender to the reality of my circumstances, the fight for a well-lived life, the wrestling with God never stops.

When nothing else seems to ease the pain, many of my students find solace in an exercise based on an ancient prayer practice that involves an almost literal "wrestling" with God.

To do this exercise, find a private space, follow your breath for a few seconds, and begin speaking out loud to whatever higher power you wish to connect with, engaging as much of your body as you can. The important thing is to take your time and stay impeccably present to whatever rises up in you. When you feel that you're veering away from the truth, stop, drop back into the heart, and begin speaking again.

Diane, a client who had gone through five years of treatments, described how one day in the middle of the exercise she suddenly found herself with fists raised and her face turned toward the heavens. "This is simply not acceptable!" she cried. "I don't know what you're thinking, but this will just not do!!!"

"It scared me," she said later, laughing a little. "The nuns at my Catholic school would've keeled over if they'd seen me carrying on like that. "

The exercise helped Diane realize that she was not quite ready to turn away from the idea of a biological child and look into other options. A few days later she found herself spontaneously repeating prayers from her childhood, something she had not done in years.

One night about a month after her face-off with God, the phone rang and I picked it up, wondering who was calling so late. "I just couldn't wait till morning, and it's much too soon, I know, I'm only about five minutes pregnant, but I just had to call!" said Diane, catching her breath.

I wish I could tell you that this is the way things turn out every time: You hurl a bucket of tears toward heaven and the next day you got mail. Not quite the way it works. Though one thing that is pretty fool proof about this prayer practice is that it can help you let go of a lifeload of pain.

How, then, do we continue to see the miraculous in all
of creation? What is it that can help us defend our faith,
and wade against the current of doubt coursing through us?
"Traditiiiiioooon...tradition!" bellows a chorus of ancestors
along a multitude of spiritual paths.

"If you're looking for allies, don't you want to clasp the
hands of those who came before you?" they intone. "Wouldn't
it make supreme sense to want to keep our stories alive; to
offer them as an invitation to the unborn; an invitation not
only on your own behalf but on behalf of all the generations
before you? The child you're heading toward is, after all, a
continuation of our story."

Our sages teach that we are born, biologically or spiri-
tually, through adoption or through any other process, into
a culture that best suits our soul's earthly mission. This
wisdom tradition is mother's milk for the soul, and no bio-
identical substitute can take its place. A Gaelic lullaby, the
beat of the djembe drums, the fire of a merengue rhythm
will set your cells in motion in a particular way. Your great-
grandmother's stories will find the hidden passageway to
your deepest Self the way nothing else will.

Sadly, many of us refuse the most nourishing morsels
of our cultural and spiritual inheritance, maybe because we
are trying to fit in, or maybe because some priest or rabbi
or nun had once served up a leathery, hard-to-swallow cut
of dogma. When we do that – when we, as Kabir says, "turn
away and walk into the dark alone," – something remains
incomplete inside us. A contact with something precious
and irreplaceable will never be made. Our inheritance remains unclaimed, like acres of soil that lie fallow with nothing planted and no hope of harvest.

Placing my story within the greater context of my an-
cestral line was not an easy task for me. I arrived in America at the age of nineteen resolved to immediately dive into

Jewish learning. Yet somehow, over thirty years of living in New York City, I could never seem to find a Hebrew literacy class that matched my schedule.

The Judaism I was raised with was a Judaism of devastation. Our once thriving Jewish community was reduced to a handful of families, each with its own legacy of losses. The majestic structure of the synagogue where we attended High Holiday services, with its rows of vacant pews, and its peeling paint, seemed to be caving in on itself, as if the weight of memory was too much for the ancient walls to bear.

So it's not surprising that my efforts to learn what being Jewish, or "doing Jewish," is all about met with repeated self-sabotage. Still I stayed the course. Over and over I heaved my climbing rope over the cliff of resistance, until one day it hooked onto the rock and I began my ascent. These days the climb is more thrilling than I could ever have imagined. I'm part of an extraordinary Jewish spiritual community. The High Holidays I attend take place in a giant white tent filled with women and men and children of all ages. I weep and chant and study the stories my mother grew up with that were too difficult for her to share with me. My library is filled with books of Hasidic Tales, and sacred text commentaries. The words of these books nourish me the way green leafy vegetables began to bring vitality back into my body fourteen years ago. Often I feast on them late into the night. My knowledge of Hebrew is still in its most rudimentary stages, and I struggle to translate the prayers I chant. But as I wrap my tongue around the sound, it vibrates and whirs and carries me across the abyss of time, and I feel my grandfather's wide open palms blessing me.

My life grew out of the ashes of World War II in 1949. My daughter Adira was born in April of '94. To some that inversion is nothing but a meaningless coincidence. To me those numbers are a teaching of the Great Reversal, part of the call all of us humans are asked to heed: the call to keep turning our curses into blessings. As much as I love getting birth announcements and photographs of new families, the most exciting part of my work is witnessing the metamorphosis that happens when someone begins to heed this call.

On my desk sit the photographs of two extraordinary women, each of them with a child in her arms. I've had the great honor to be a part of Monica's and Hannah's stories for three years, much longer than I usually get to actively participate in people's journeys. During that time I've seen these two courageous women walk over countless bridges of fear, frustration, grief, and loss. And each time I watched them land safely on the other side of the bridge and get right back on the trail. Monica's daughter, Anna, arrived after a full-term pregnancy and Hannah's son, Russian-born Sasha, arrived in America in the arms of his two adoring parents. What these two women had in common was that they both seized the opportunity of their crisis and didn't let go. They kept reaching out and walking toward their child until one day they found their child reaching out for them..

In a recent note Hannah writes:

> *I can't help but think of the first workshop I attended and an imagery exercise about what I would need to pack for my journey towards my child. I remember thinking of the child far away and stretching out their arms to me. The funny thing is that Sasha loves to lunge and stretch out towards me - out of reach... he giggles uncontrollably and then runs towards me at full speed. I think he must know how much we longed for him, he seems to have longed for*

*us too. He is so happy, we are so happy – so full
of joy – I just can't believe it".*

If only we could trust the great Bestower of Babies to
know just what to do; to deliver the cherished child on our
doorstep the same way it once delivered us. If only we could
trust that this Awarder of Babies makes no mistakes, that
it grants each of us who stay the course the perfect baby, a
perfect match, a perfect teacher. One who will challenge us
in the precise manner that suits our soul. If only we could
trust that it is bound to happen if we keep our arms open
to receive, and don't stop until we feel the baby's weight
against our chest.

Everything we do becomes a thousand times more
meaningful if it's an expression of our trust, sent out as a
prayer in action. Every ounce of vegetable juice, every yoga
posture, every imagery exercise then becomes an act of surrender. It's a way of saying that we're willing to do whatever
it takes to meet God and this baby halfway. My students
sometimes ask, "But what about all those people who prac-
tically bathe in caffeine and live on candy bars and pop out
one kid after another? What about them?" The best answer
I've come up with so far is that we all have our own divinely
tailored assignment, our own heroic mission to fulfill. We
don't know what someone else's mission might be.

After September 11, a Native American grandfather
was explaining to his grandson how he felt about the tragedy. "I feel as though I have two wolves fighting in my heart,"
he said. "One wolf wants revenge and the other wants to
understand, and to stop this from ever happening again."

"And which wolf will win the fight in your heart?" the
boy asked.

"The one I feed, " replied the grandfather.

At any given point throughout this journey, two birds

might sing in your head. The bird of doubt sings the song of blame and misfortune and self-flagellation. The bird of faith says, "More shall be revealed." You'll have to decide which of those two birds you choose to feed.

Chapter 11
The Not-Yet-Born

"Lack of awareness of the basic unity of organism and environment is a serious and dangerous hallucination. For in a civilization equipped with immense technological power, the sense of alienation between man and nature leads to the use of technology in a hostile spirit..."

– Alan Watts,
Psychedelics and Religious Experience

In an ancient village torn apart by war, starvation, and disease, a circle of women gathered in prayer. "What shall we pray for?" one woman asked. "Our sons are dying in battle: shall we pray for the war to end?" "Our children are hungry," said another. "We must pray for a bountiful harvest." "Our mothers are weak with fever," wailed the youngest. "Let's pray for a medicine to bring them relief." "No, my child," spoke the village wise woman, her voice barely a whisper. "We cannot pray to end war, for we have already been given a human heart to help us find peace within ourselves and with our neighbors. If only we would use it. We cannot pray to end starvation, for we have already been given the soil to grow enough food to feed the whole world. If only we would use it with care. We cannot pray to end disease, for we have already been given the wisdom to find healing for everything that ails us. If only we would use it." A breeze moved in from the ocean, and the wise woman said, "Sweet sisters, let's pray for humility and determination." The old matriarch's face was bathed in sunlight as she cleared her throat and bowed her head. "Let's pray for strength to live our prayers."

– Story inspired by a prayer service led by Gershon Winkler

On a morning news show, a woman in her early thirties speaks of abating her fears of childlessness by freezing her eggs. Later, I receive an invitation to support an education campaign, launched by pharmaceutical companies and in vitro fertilization clinics, that aims to inform the public about advances in treatments. At a luncheon a couple bemoans the fact that their insurance covers only three in vitro cycles.

"Our friends in Boston qualified for an over-forty study sponsored by their clinic and the National Institute of Health. They've been approved for *six* in-vitro cycles; the first four have failed but they have two more to go," says the husband.

The very same evening, a colleague comes across a report on the rising ratio of Japanese babies conceived through technology, and a press release:

"US Researcher Working on Artificial Womb."

I listen and read and can't help thinking that something is being omitted: the piece of the puzzle that would turn "infertility" into a "lesson-in-fertility."

Medical technology can be a wonderful, immensely powerful tool. It harms or heals us, depending on how we use it.

I wonder if anyone who has worked in the field of reproductive health in any capacity would argue with the notion that a road paved with hormone stimulants ought to bear a flashing sign: "Proceed with Caution!" Though some of the routinely prescribed drugs now do display a similar warning, it's an advisory which I see repeatedly disregarded. When we use technology to silence the pleading voices within us, and assault our bodies with increasingly more potent protocols, an instrument of healing becomes a dangerous, self-punishing weapon.

The manner in which my doctors delivered their diagnosis and prognosis fifteen years ago was hurtful. But looking back, I'm grateful that they categorically refused to further traumatize my tottering endocrine system.

Someday an artificial womb might become a simple childbearing option. Today, achieving a healthy pregnancy is still one of the medical challenges where certainty eludes even the best and the brightest. The most hard-core scientist will admit that a feisty follicle and a spunky sperm do not necessarily a baby make. Something about conceiving a life makes it startlingly clear that we are more than a collection of well-designed organs. To participate in it consciously requires an honest commitment to oneself, to another human being, and to some mystery that breathes within the world.

"The not-yet-born, who still know everything" is a phrase from Mary Oliver's poem "In Blackwater Woods." I wonder what the not-yet-born are trying to tell us these days. If I were a silky-faced baby about to plunge into this world, I would unquestionably lobby for change. A radical change.

What if the unborn have launched an education campaign of their own, and the growing number of couples with reproductive challenges is part of their strategic plan? Perhaps somewhere in the overworld a council of babies-to-be convenes each day, a council whose mission is to create a more child-friendly planet. Perhaps the members of this council have vetoed breast milk laced with heavy metals and gasoline as an acceptable food item. Chances are they've been briefed about endocrine disruptors such as dioxin – the most poisonous organic man-made chemical, second in toxicity only to radioactive waste – and know that these are not only slowing down our sperm and confusing our pituitary gland; are not only killing off species of butterflies, birds, fish, beetles, and bees; aren't just contaminating the water, food, and air *we* breathe. They're destroying the resources our children will need to live.

Perhaps the not-yet-born are becoming seriously worried.

Last night my older daughter Ellena lined up at the Golden Notebook, a bookstore in town, to buy her copy of the latest Harry Potter novel. My husband tells me he saw a man in a business suit carrying a copy of the book under his arm as he boarded the early morning commuter train. Ten million copies of *Harry Potter and the Half-Blood Prince* were bought on the first day it went on sale. We, adults and children alike, are rooting for the boy who is destined to redeem his world from evil. If only for the short time of our daily commute, we yearn to live in the world of magic. We want to be reassured that what we see is not all there is, that somewhere a parallel universe exists, with its own language and inhabitants of astonishing powers, where life is one breathless adventure after another. A land where justice prevails and evil is defeated.

I say a world like that does exist, though right now the outline of it is but a faint mark on the canvas of our imagination. There are many who will tell you that such a world is inconceivable. Cruelty, corruption, and betrayal, they'll say, are part of human nature.

You and I can conjure up countless stories to justify our complacency. I'm ashamed to admit this, but for many years I thought of myself as being apolitical. At the time, it was the best defense I could muster for feeling utterly powerless. Today I know that there is no such thing as being apolitical. To be alive is to stand for something. We can choose wholeheartedly what it is we want to stand for or let someone else choose instead, but the ground we stand on is not a neutral zone.

Growing up as I did with stories of grandmothers, aunts, and cousins who, had they not been murdered, would have loved me *oh so much*, the desire that dominated my child-hood daydreams was a desire for family. Soon after I came to America, in a time that was very lonely, I would sit on the subway or the bus, and all the faces around me would look vaguely familiar. It felt as though we were all distant relatives who no longer recognized one another, no longer remembered our common origin. Sometimes I'd fantasize about tearful reunions, followed by holiday feasts with a large, noisy, extended family.

I got my wish, though it didn't quite happen as I imagined it would. I'm no longer alone, not only because I have a husband and children and friends, but because today I feel closely related to everyone who yearns for a healthy, peaceful world and is willing to do what it takes to birth it. To conceive it, nurture its gestation, embrace the labor pain of every contraction, and brace for the great push to bring it forth. The women and men who in spite of all evidence to the contrary, insist on changing the world are my family: my grandmothers, my uncles and aunts, my brothers and sisters.

Those of us who have faced difficulties in our desire to parent a child make up a global community. How that community will affect the world health care system, econ-omy, agriculture, peace efforts, and human consciousness depends on how each of us meets the roadblocks in our way.

It's Labor Day weekend, and on Tuesday Ellena and Adi start school again. We'll walk to the corner in the morn-ing. They'll climb the steps of the school bus and go off into a world that appears to be more dangerous every day. There is nowhere to run, or hide. It's no use pretending that there is anything that happens anywhere on the planet that isn't happening to every one of us. And when it's the apple of your heart's eye you send out into the world each day, the stakes suddenly shoot way up.

I'd like to think that our lesson in fertility is a lesson in usefulness. I imagine the unborn, as well as the children who are already here, pleading with us to speak up on their behalf: to begin to nurture ourselves, one another, and the earth as tenderly as we yearn to care for them.

My fervent desire is that, by the time you reach this page, you will have realized that the power to change your life and the world is in your hands. If bringing a vision of a healthy, peaceful planet into physical reality is not at the top of the list of every human hoping to parent a child, then we have missed the point. And missed a momentous opportunity. I pray that this book might in a small way insure that that does not happen. After all, a longing is a terrible thing to waste.

Part Four

Fertile Heart™ Ovum Practice

Chapter 12

Practice, Practice, Practice

"I follow my protocol religiously...wouldn't dream of missing a day...I need to show my body I can be counted on."

– from *Inconceivable*

Remember the old joke? A man walking up Broadway in his best concert attire stops an elderly woman.

"Excuse me," he asks, "how do I get to Carnegie Hall?"

She looks at him with a wise, steady gaze and says:

"Practice, practice, practice!"

The essence of the Fertile Heart practice is spending quality time with the child already here, our own body, heart, and soul, and discovering what truly nourishes us. Not what we're addicted to, or what we use to numb our pain or distract ourselves, but what it is that truly feeds us.

The chapters in this section are meant to be an invitation rather than a prescription; a sharing of the carefully crafted tools I have continued to use in my own ongoing birthing practice, tools that have been useful to the thousands of women and men I've had the privilege to work with. At the same time, in order for them to become medicinal, a degree of steadfastness is necessary. If you reach for them once in a while, as the mood strikes you, they will become just another item on your to-do-list. They may make you feel happy, or hopeful, for a day or so, but ultimately not much will come of them. If, however, you respect them and treat them as powerful remedies, they're bound to become agents of change on every level.

After you've worked with the tools in this section for a couple of weeks, you may want to go back and reread the corresponding chapters. The deeper your understanding of what it is you're attempting to do, the more valuable the tools will be for you.

The suggestions offered here are meant to free you, so that you can live your longing with more passion and curiosity and awe than you have ever done before. And above all, don't keep looking down at your feet to make sure you're doing it right. Just turn up the music and dance!

Chapter 13

Fertile Heart™ Imagery

"I had so many emotional scars, it was scary for me to delve into the invisible stuff. But when I started to do the imagery daily, things really began to change and I felt a weight lifting off my shoulders."

– Fertile Heart workshop participant

If dreams are letters from God, consistent imaging work is our way of keeping up our end of the correspondence, and deepening our relationship with the ineffable. For just about every one of the women I worked with, imagery was an essential element of their self-healing protocol.

Here are a few suggestions on the "when and how" of this practice. Ideally you should do the exercise of your choice twice a day, in the morning as soon as you wake up, and in the evening shortly before you go to bed. It is recommended that you sit with your spine straight and begin each sequence of images by articulating an intention; reminding and clarifying to yourself what you hope to resolve with this particular imaginal remedy.

The next step is to close your eyes and allow the breath to move through you for a few seconds without manipulating it in any way. When you feel grounded and ready to move on, reverse your habitual way of breathing by focusing on the exhalation. In other words, begin each breath with a long slow exhalation through the mouth, then inhale through the nose. The longer and slower the exhalation, the deeper the imagery experience. Do this reverse breathing three or four times before each exercise, until you feel ready to move on to imaging. By changing your breathing you give yourself a signal that you are changing your ordinary, mechanical way of being in the world. You're giving yourself a subliminal message that change is possible.

The deliberate focus on the out-breath is, for me, also a

reminder that we are breathing life into these new images. You conclude each visualization with one long outbreath.

Whatever imagery you choose to work with, I recommend that you do each one for cycles of seven, fourteen, or twenty-one days. In the course of each cycle the images might change, evolve, bring new messages and new insights, or remain unchanged. Try to see the images that rise up as additional clues, information to be used in whatever way you find most appropriate.

The one thing that stops most of us from learning something new is comparing it with something we've learned or heard about before. The Fertile Heart way of working with pictures engages your will and creativity in a manner that is quite specific and different from the more familiar style of visualizations. So to get the full value of the medicine, I encourage you to read through the "Image by Image" chapter a few times and to follow the above instructions for at least a few months before making any adjustments to your practice. The Fertile Heart Imagery CD, and Fertile Heart Imagery 2 CD, offer additional guidance along with fifty two imaginal remedies to support you in meeting your child halfway.

(A "New Beginning" was inspired by one of Colette Aboulker-Muscat's exercises.)

A New Beginning

Intention:

To clear away all that does not serve you and prepare the ground for a new beginning.

Close your eyes, observe your breath for a few seconds, then breathe out three times with long, slow exhalations.

See yourself at the seashore, fully clothed and heading toward the water. As you move forward, you are removing your articles of clothing one at a time. You empty your pockets, bag, or purse, keeping only what's indispensable. Once you're naked, you make an abrasive compound from sand and water and clean yourself thoroughly from head to toe. When you finish cleaning yourself on the outside, clean yourself inside – of despair, gloom, beliefs about age, statistics, pessimism, confusion.

Dive into the sea, immersing yourself fully, and cleaning off any residue with sand from the bottom of the sea.

When you are finished, let the sun dry you off.

Lying on the sand, find a brand new set of clothing.

The River of Truth

Intention:

If you're wrestling with questions about treatment options or any other aspect of your journey, this exercise can encourage an answer to rise up. (Also see the "Fork in the Road" exercise in the "Image by Image" chapter.)

Close your eyes, observe your breath for a few seconds, then breathe out three times with long, slow exhalations.

See yourself standing on a riverbank. This is the River of Truth.

Breathe out once and cast a golden fishing line into the water. See and sense the current pulling your line.

Breathe out once.

When you feel the answer attach to the fishing line, begin to slowly reel it in. Receive the answer you retrieved in whatever form it has been delivered.

Breathe out and open your eyes.

Repeat the exercise until the answer is clear. The exercise might also encourage "guiding dreams" that are specific to the question you posed.

The Backpack

Intention:

To reach clarity about all the missing pieces of your life, pieces that perhaps a part of you expects the baby to fill.

Close your eyes, observe your breath for a few seconds, then breathe out three times with long, slow exhalations.

See yourself standing at the foot of a mountain, waiting. In your pocket, find a pair of silver binoculars. Use them to look toward the top of the mountain, where your baby is preparing for her/his journey to you. The baby's body is weighed down by a heavy backpack. It is filled with all that you expect motherhood to bring you. With your binoculars you can see the entire contents of the backpack. You might see such items as self-esteem, forgiveness, and success.

Breathe out once.

Know, sense, and feel that you do not need to depend on the baby to deliver any of these items to you, that you can find a way to create them for yourself. Now see a pair of hands gently remove the backpack from the baby and hurl it off into the distance, where it's washed away by a giant waterfall.

Your child is now free to set out on the journey without excess luggage.

Breathe out and open your eyes.

Retrieving the Treasure

Intention:

To receive guidance about the next step in your pilgrimage.

Close your eyes, observe your breath for a few seconds, then breathe out three times with long slow exhalations.

Dive into the deepest part of you and on the ocean floor of your heart's truth find a case. What does it look like?

Breathe out once.

Swim back up to the surface with the case. Open the case. What have you found? How does this image provide the next clue? How can you use it to strengthen and nourish you?

The Ropes of Obligation

Intention:

To separate your Orphan rooted desire for a child from the yearning of the Visionary mother within you.

Close your eyes, breathe out three times with long slow exhalations.

Invite an image of a woman held hostage in an isolated place, bound with heavy ropes. Attached to the ropes is a sign: "You must have a biological child or else..." (complete the sentence each time you do the exercise). See yourself step inside the image with a pair of large golden scissors. With the next breath cut the ropes and attend to the woman's wounds. Take a silver jar filled with the salve of compassion and unconditional kindness, and apply it to any part of her body where the ropes may have cut into the flesh.

Breathe out and open your eyes.

The Glass House

Intention:

To unravel the underlying truth of difficult feelings; to take care of the Inner Orphan asking to be heard. (After you've done this exercise for a few days, you may want to invite your Inner Orphan and your Ultimate Mom to articulate their feelings in form of a letter. Pouring your heart out on paper can be powerful medicine.)

Close your eyes, observe your breath for a few seconds, then breathe out three times with long, slow exhalations.

See and sense yourself standing in front of a house made of glass. You are able to see everything that happens inside. Give yourself permission to fully experience all that you are feeling at this moment.

Breathe out once.

Now look directly in front of you and see, in one of the rooms of the glass house, a child who feels exactly the way you are feeling at this moment. The child is you at age ___ (Allow the image to rise up, the age of the child might change each time you do the exercise.)

Notice articles of the child's clothing, including their colors, and the objects in the room. Let the child express all that she needs to express as fully as possible, through her voice, and her entire body.

Breathe out once.

If there are other people in the house who should be part of this scene, let them come in. See if there is anything that needs to be said, or done.

Breathe out once.

Now invite an image of yourself as an adult entering the scene. Ask yourself, Is this adult an Orphan, or a Visionary mom?

Breathe out once.

If there is anything you wish to do or say to anyone, do so as fully and clearly as you can. If you'd like to comfort the child, do so in any way that feels appropriate.

Whenever you are ready, say good-bye, and know that you can return to this house anytime you wish.

Breathe out and open your eyes.

Authority

Intention:

To become your own authority.

Close your eyes, observe your breath for a few seconds, then breathe out three times with long, slow exhalations.

See, sense, and feel yourself standing in the Field of Creation. Your body is grounded in the earth, nourished by the multitude of underground roots spread across the field. On the left side of the field, invite the images of the false authorities in your life.

Breathe out once.

With the next inhalation, see a power line extending from your body to each of the authorities. Ask yourself if you wish to continue supplying these voices with energy.

Breathe out once.

Choose to cut the power line with a pair of giant gold scissors.

Breathe out once.

See a current of pure water clear the field of any debris. The Field of Creation is now free of false voices.

Breathe out once.

Invite the image of one true voice of authority that supports your highest good and well being. Welcome this voice and offer your gratitude for the guidance it gives you.

The Pillow

Intention:

To let go of the past and open up to creation.

Close your eyes, observe your breath for a few seconds, then breathe out three times with long, slow exhalations.

See yourself sitting in your home, holding a pillow. Notice what you're wearing, where you're sitting, and the texture and color of the pillow. Hold on to the pillow as tightly as you wish. Sewn into this pillow is all the accumulated suffering, abuse, violence, and loss that you and members of your family have gone through, in your generation as well as in the generations before you.

Breathe out once.

Ask yourself whether or not you're willing to let go of this pillow. Answer truthfully. Breathe out again, and choose to let go.

As you do this, see the windows and doors of your home open, and see and feel a breeze and a golden light pour into the house. Let your arms open and see the pillow be lifted and carried off through the open windows behind you.

Know that it is your choice to let go that has transformed the pillow of suffering into an energy of light and life.

Breathe out again and feel your open arms and body ready to receive the guidance of the Ultimate Mom and conceive all that asks to be birthed through you.

Breathe out and open your eyes.

Motherhood Revised

Intention:

To release Orphan-rooted beliefs about motherhood and parenting.

Close your eyes, observe your breath for a few seconds, then breathe out three times with long, slow exhalations.

Invite an image of yourself as a child with your mother.

Breathe out once.

See your mother during a difficult moment.

Breathe out once.

Allow the experience of the image to move through you. Ask yourself: Is this the kind of mother I want to be?

Breathe out once.

Invite an image of yourself and your child. How are you similar to your mom; how are you different?

Know, sense, and feel at the deepest level of your being that you have the inner resources to become the Visionary mother you wish to be.

Breathe out and open your eyes.

You may want to do the same exercise inviting an image of yourself with your father.

The White Ribbon

Intention:

To stop recurrent pregnancy loss, and to realize that each pregnancy is the start of a new life.

Close your eyes, observe your breath for a few seconds, then breathe out three times with long, slow exhalations.

See a white, flowing ribbon. Take a pair of golden scissors and cut the ribbon into three separate pieces, each of a different length. Know, sense, and feel that as each piece of the ribbon is separate from the next, each child that comes into the world comes with her/his own message and her/his own unique purpose.

Breathe out and open your eyes.

Cell Talk

Intention:

To deepen your trust in the Ultimate Mom wisdom weaved into every cell of your Holy Human Loaf.

Close your eyes, observe your breath for a few seconds, then breathe out three times with long, slow exhalations.

Invite an image of yourself inside your body. You're standing in a place from which you can easily communicate with every cell.

Let the breath move through you and listen. What do you hear? Is there a cluster of cells that calls for your attention? Is there anything you want to ask or say to the cells of your body?

Breathe out once.

Scan your body and find a cluster of cells that knows that making a baby is not a very difficult assignment. Listen to them speak. Invite all of your bodymind to hear what they have to say.

Breathe out once.

Is there anything else you wish to ask or communicate?

Breathe out once.

Thank the cells for their confidence.

Breathe out and open your eyes.

Orchard of Possibilities

Intention:

To identify obstacles that stop you from becoming pregnant and receive guidance for your particular healing regimen.

Close your eyes, observe your breath for a few seconds, then breathe out three times with long, slow exhalations.

Invite an image of a road leading to an orchard. A plaque on the gate reads: "Orchard of Possibilities." You find a key to open the gate and step inside the stone enclosure. On the right you see an ancient tree offering shade and protection. You sit cross-legged leaning against the tree, and look down at your belly. It is full of life; you are in your last trimester of pregnancy. Place your hand on your belly and feel the movement of the baby.

Breathe out once.

Ask yourself: What was it that made this pregnancy possible? What made a difference? Let the breath move through you, and let the answer rise up of its own accord. (It might be a different answer each time you do the exercise, or there might be times when no answer comes. Be patient.)

Breathe out once.

Stand up and walk over to the birthing tree standing in the far corner of the orchard. Your partner or friends are waiting there for you with a blanket. The branches of the tree bend over you protectively. The tree and the entire orchard are there to support and strengthen you for the birthing of your new baby. With the next breath feel the baby move through the birth canal.

See, hold, and breathe in the sweet presence of your child. Give thanks to the Bestower of Babies.

Breathe out and open your eyes. An

An Offering

Intention:

To experience your ability to ask for help without judging your feelings and thoughts as positive or negative. .

Close your eyes, observe your breath for a few seconds, then breathe out three times with long, slow exhalations.

Invite an image of a silver tray.

Breathe out once.

Without judging or censoring, invite onto the tray images that articulate all that is present for you at this moment:any feelings or thoughts.

Breathe out once.

Offer all that you have placed on the tray as your gift to the Source of Creation. Trust that everything that you offer with a pure intention is instantly transformed into a life-enhancing instrument of healing.

Breathe out and open your eyes.

Blanket of Reassurance

Intention:

To enhance your trust in the Ultimate Mom wisdom that governs the growth of your child.

Close your eyes, observe your breath for a few seconds, then breathe out three times with long, slow exhalations.

Invite an image of a large soft blanket. Know that all that has been good, and wise has been woven into it by the generations of women who came before you. Only their love and their deepest truth is carried in the delicate threads of your blanket. As you wrap it around you, you can feel their guidance inscribed in every cell of your body, and in the growing body of your child.

Breathe out and open your eyes.

Without judging or censoring, invite onto the tray images that articulate all that is present for you at this moment:any feelings or thoughts.

Breathe out once.

Offer all that you have placed on the tray as your gift to the Source of Creation. Trust that everything that you offer with a pure intention is instantly transformed into a life-enhancing instrument of healing.

Breathe out and open your eyes.

Trusting the Bestower

Intention:

Deepening our understanding of the difference between "giving up" on our desire and surrendering to the Ultimate Mom wisdom that guides our human choices at all times.

Invite an image of a sacred protected space, governed by the Bestower of Babies. See the vegetation in this place, the colors, the weather.

Breathe out once

Invite an image of the Bestower of Babies. Allow the image to rise up into your field of inner vision.

See yourself and your partner with the baby in your arms. The baby that you feel should be in your arms at this moment. Receive the presence of the child, the sweet fran-grance, the silky smooth skin.

Breathe out once.

Ask yourself "Do I trust that the Bestower of Babies is on my side?" Let the truth of the moment rise up without judging.

With the next breath see yourself entrusting the baby in your arms to the Bestower.

Breathe out once and know that this act of surrender is a giant step toward meeting your child halfway in physical reality.

Chapter 14

Fertile Heart™
Dream-Reading Practice

"I have never been able to visualize my child, in the past the only image that would come was me as a child. But last night I saw her! She was a year old, with curly black hair, and dark eyes. She exuded a calm, sweet energy."

– Fertile Heart workshop participant

The first thing to do is to buy a gorgeous journal to keep next to your bed, and a small flashlight for occasional mid-sleep notes. (Some people feel that a tape recorder captures a mood of the dream more vividly.) Before you go to bed, open the journal and write: Dream of.....and the following day's date. As you drift off to sleep, say to yourself: I remember my dreams and I write them down when I wake up.

Even if you never remember your dreams, consistent imagery practice will help change that. Be patient. If all you're left with in the morning is a vague sense of an image, or a feeling you can't quite identify, take a few minutes and try to describe your experience. Usually, the act of writing things down will jolt your memory.

It is, of course, best to record your dream in as much detail as you can, as soon as you first open your eyes in the morning. But if that's not possible, jot down a few images or some key words and at some point during the day or that evening go back and fill in the rest.

In the next few pages I'll share examples of pivotal dream sequences of ten of my students, and the insights they gleaned as they worked with particular dream-reading questions. Sometimes the revelations unfolded gradually through discussion, or simply by letting the dream simmer on a back burner of their awareness. When we are caught up in a conflict or a difficulty, every dream comes to offer additional clues. Since the desire to become a mother was the main focus in each of these women's lives, we looked at each dream sequence as a guidepost in their pilgrimage, even if on the surface the dream seemed unrelated to the baby search.

Some people like to give their dreams a title, such as one might give a short story. If you find that it's helpful, go ahead and do that, though you may want to contemplate the images for a while before choosing a title. For me, naming dreams limits the decoding process.

To review, here are the basic questions we work with:

– **What is the strongest feeling in the dream?** Is there an image that evokes an intense emotional reaction? Is it a feeling I'm not ordinarily aware of, one of my Inner Orphans calling for attention? Why is the Dream Teacher asking me to engage with it at this juncture in my pilgrimage?

– **What is the strongest feeling I have after waking up?** Is it different from the feeling in the dream? Is this feeling revealing an Orphan or allowing me to experience more directly the Visionary part of me?

– **How is the dream or any part of it similar to circumstances in my waking reality?** Is the dream inviting a new way of seeing those circumstances?

– **Is the dream validating or rejecting a choice I've made in my waking life?**

– **What direction is the dream moving in?** Who am I at the beginning, and who am I at the end of the dream? The Dream Teacher might be pointing us in a direction of growth, and this question can help us recognize what that direction is.

– **If someone I know appears in the dream, why is**

he/she showing up right now? In what way am I behaving like this person? What is this person's most pronounced character trait? The dream might be letting me know that this trait is a part of me, and I need to become aware of it.

Read the dream again, and see every person or animal or object in the dream as an expression of you. Ask yourself what their various characteristics are and why they are being called to your attention at this point. You may want to experiment with "sensing" what it would feel like to become that person, or animal, or object. How would you move? What would you sound like?

Understand that each dream is an invitation to change something in your waking life, an attitude, belief, or behavior. What are you being asked to change this time?

In the dream reading examples that follow, we worked through each sequence and the dreamer and I chose one or more of the above questions to initiate the reading. Sometimes the insights arose instantly, and sometimes they unfolded in the days or weeks after our initial exploration.

Maria's Dream

Many of my students have important guiding dreams after they register to attend a workshop. Maria lives on the West Coast. A trip to Woodstock was a major investment of money, time, and effort.

> *"I am in the small town where I was born, and where my father had a sporting goods store. He is closing the store because a war is about to start. I am angry and say to him: 'Why do we need to get involved in another war? We don't care who wins or loses; the result is the same. Why don't you tell them to leave us alone, we just want to work!' My*

father says: "That is not true, Maria. It doesn't matter if you lose or win, but you have to fight for what you believe in.'"

Is the dream validating or rejecting a choice I've made in my waking life?

"I was really struggling to figure out if I should go through all the trouble and expense of the trip to Woodstock, and even after I registered I wasn't sure I was really going to make it. It was the dream that made me finally make up my mind. The story made even more sense after the workshop. 'Business as usual' was definitely over, and I had to get out there and fight a war, mostly a war with myself, with the part of me that doesn't feel that what I do makes a bit of difference."

Read the dream again, and see every person or animal or object in the dream as an expression of you. Ask yourself what their various characteristics are and why they are being called to your attention. You may want to experiment with "sensing" what it would feel like to become that person, or animal, or object. How would you move? What would you sound like?

"My father has always been one of my heroes; he is someone who will speak up for the truth no matter what. The dream is letting me know that my father's integrity and courage are part of me. It's time to speak up, to start advocating for myself."

Cynthia's Dream

A common theme for many of the women I work with is a feeling of inadequacy, of not being able to take care of a child, of inadvertently harming her/him. There are countless reasons for such feelings, among them: being poorly cared for as a child; unfelt rage; fear of not meeting your own or other people's expectations.

"I'm with the baby, and I realize I don't know how to feed her. The baby slips out of my hand and bangs her head against the table, and it looks like her eyes are rolling over in her head. I tell myself that if she dies, I won't tell anyone."

What is the strongest feeling I have after waking up? Is it different from the feeling in the dream?

"I was scared when I saw the baby's eyes rolling over in her head, but in the dream I was kind of matter-of-fact about hiding it. That was shocking to me when I read through it in the morning. As I worked with the images, and thought of myself as the baby in the dream, what came to me is that I've become pretty matter-of-fact about hiding the 'little murders' of my own soul. I was a pretty lonely child and a wild, rebellious teenager, and I kept a lot hidden from my parents."

How is the dream or any part of it similar to circumstances in my waking reality? Is the dream inviting a new way of seeing those circumstances?

"I'm definitely nervous about taking care of a baby, but I have friends who have children, and I can get help. What

I think is more urgent is learning how to feed myself. I'm
the baby whose head's been 'banged against the table' over
and over again, especially since we started trying to get
pregnant. I really don't want to do that anymore."

Lynn's Dream

> *"I was in a kind of a cathedral but it had no ceil-*
> *ing, just these very high, majestical walls. It was*
> *full of people, and they were singing a hymn. I*
> *couldn't recognize the language, but it sounded*
> *familiar. I was trying to find a place to sit. I*
> *wanted to sit up front and there was an empty*
> *seat there but I decided to walk to the back."*

What is the strongest feeling in the dream? Is there
an image that evokes an intense emotional reaction? Is it
a feeling I'm not ordinarily aware of, one of my Inner Orphans calling for attention? Why is the Dream Teacher asking me to engage with it at this juncture in my pilgrimage?

"I was grieving my third miscarriage, working with the
glass house imagery for about two weeks on my own and
in the group, when this dream came. So I was surprised
to realize that the strongest feeling in the dream was joy.
Almost overwhelming joy. The images were very spacious
and full of light; it made me feel very hopeful."

Read the dream again, and see every person or animal
or object in the dream as an expression of you. Ask yourself what their various characteristics are and why they
are being called to your attention at this point. You may
want to experiment with "sensing" what it would feel like
to become that person, or animal, or object. How would you

move? What would you sound like?

"What struck me was that the cathedral had no ceiling. And the walls were made of very light transparent material. I've been pretty stoic about my miscarriages; I haven't even told my best friend about them. It feels like the dream is telling me that I need to let people see what is inside me, that I need to reach out to people."

Understand that each dream is an invitation to change something in your waking life, an attitude, belief, or behavior. What are you being asked to change this time?

"I was happy to hear the singing, but I was also unsure where my seat was, how I belonged to these people. The dream was telling me that I had to 'find my seat.' My mother was Welsh; she died a few years ago, but I have a vague memory of her singing to us when my brother and I were very small. Hearing the hymn was comforting. I need to somehow find a place for myself in the community I came from. My husband and I don't belong to any church. He is really down on organized religion, but I think we both need to be part of some sort of spiritual community. We just have to find one that's right for us."

Alice's Dream

"I'm in my house and it's very comfortable and safe there, but when I look out the window I see that I'm in a land that I'm not familiar with. The land I live on has been conquered by a nation. As long as I stay in my house I'm safe, but when I step outside I'm a slave."

How is the dream or any part of it similar to circumstances in my waking reality? Is the dream inviting a new way of seeing those circumstances?

"I've become a slave to the obsession to have a baby. This obsession is controlling me and I've become enslaved by it. I need to change that. Also, I am always searching the different fertility sites, asking people about their protocols, and it's exhausting me. The dream is telling me to stay in my own house. My body is my house; I carry it around wherever I go. If I stay in the house, I'll be safe; if I can just stay home – in my body – I'll be safe."

Julie's Recurring Dream

Many of my students have recurring dreams about precious jewels being stolen or lost.

> *"I have a recurring dream that my jewels are stolen, and I'm in a panic, thinking: How could I let this happen? It's very real. I wake up with this terrible feeling of something being stolen from me because of my own carelessness."*

Read the dream again, and see every person, or animal or object in the dream as an expression of you. Ask yourself what are the characteristics of that person, animal or object and why are they being called to your attention at this point. The dream might be letting you know that that character trait is part of you and you need to own it. You may want to experiment with "sensing" what it would feel like to become that person, animal or object. How would you move? What would you sound like?

"When I first read this dream I thought, ' Well, of course the baby is the precious thing being taken away from me.' I didn't have a miscarriage, but I had expected to have at least two children at this stage in my life and that dream was taken away. On some level I know that that's true, but as we continued to talk about it, what really hit home was that my life was being stolen. The most precious thing is my life, and the dream was telling me that someone was stealing my life."

How is the dream or any part of it similar to circumstances in my waking reality? Is the dream inviting a new way of seeing those circumstances?

"My life was being stolen. And I was the thief. I was stealing from my time with Martin. Every minute we were together was consumed with this desperation to make a baby. We were not making love anymore; we were just failing to produce. It really hit me, when I invited the image of myself as the robber and saw myself sneaking into the house and opening cabinets and frantically grabbing everything that was valuable. It shook me up. I just said, Okay, this is it. No more shots, no more appointments, no more searching for a miracle cure. I even cancelled my acupuncture sessions. I wanted the thief to return to the scene of the crime and bring back all the jewels."

Briana's Dream

This is a dream that came several times just as Briana began ovulating. She felt guilty about dreaming of a former boyfriend and didn't bring the dream into the session for a long time. When she finally did, it turned out to be an important part of the baby puzzle. Since Briana's dream, I have often asked clients to pay close attention to dreams they have around the time of ovulation.

> *"I'm in an apartment I used to share with my former boyfriend. He is breaking up with me, telling me he can't make a commitment. He says he loves me but he is not ready to get married. I'm sobbing and throwing at him anything I can grab, until he finally walks out of the house, looking very guilty."*

Read the dream again, and see every person, or animal or object in the dream as an expression of you. Ask yourself what are the characteristics of that object and why are they being called to your attention at this point. The dream might be letting you know that that character trait is part of you and you need to own it. You may want to experiment with "sensing" what it would feel like to become that person or animal. How would you move? What would you sound like?

"I kept thinking: What in the world is this guy still doing in my dreams, I want him out. Gus, my ex-boyfriend, used to always tell me how much he cared about me, but that he just wasn't ready to make a commitment. It used to infuriate me, because he didn't want to break up, but he didn't want us to move in together or get engaged either. It looks like the dream is telling me that for all the talk of how desperately I want to have a child, there is a part of me that's like Gus. Part of me is scared to feel so much love, to make that kind of commitment to another person."

"At first it was difficult for Briana to face her "Gus nature," but the more she imaged and journaled and conversed with that part of herself, the easier it was for her to see how much her fear had thwarted her efforts not only in the baby search, but in every other part of her life.

Sheri's Dream

> *"I walk into my husband Matt's office and I see a woman in a skimpy waitress uniform standing at his desk and serving him food. He's on the phone and he absentmindedly starts picking pieces of food from the tray. He doesn't see me walk in. The waitress smiles at me, and continues to attend to Matt.*
>
> *"In the next scene Matt and I are at a medical conference and he's sitting with a bunch of his buddies from med school. I'm talking to friends of ours, a couple we know from back home who recently had their third child. They're telling me that they're opening a practice together.*
>
> *"In the last image Matt and I are walking into the operating room. We'll be performing surgery together, and all the hospital 'heavies' are there to watch."*

What direction is the dream moving in? Who am I at the beginning, and who am I at the end of the dream? (The Dream Teacher might be pointing us in a direction of growth, and this question can help us recognize what that direction is.)

"I can't say I was really feeling very much in the dream; it felt more like I was watching this movie. But when I chose the question and saw who I was in the first image and who I

~~was in the last, I started to feel more connected to my feel-~~
ings. My husband and I are both dermatologists, we have
a practice together, but since the whole baby thing started,
I've taken so much time off, I don't feel like I'm being taken
seriously by the staff or by Matt. I'm definitely more like a
waitress, constantly trying to feed him his vitamins and his
pumpkin seeds, and trying to get him to eat better.

"I don't want to be the only caretaker, I'm exhausted.
I'm in a rage when I think of having to take care of a baby
and Matt.

"The friends in the dream and the 'heavies' in the last
image are mirroring what I want right now. I want us to
become true partners, not just in the office, but at home. I
don't want to be the only one driving the whole baby thing."

In our relationships with our significant others, members of our family, or friends, it is certainly useful to realize
what it is we want from them. It is also essential for us to
work through all our difficult feelings, to recognize which
of our Inner Orphans is trying to get our attention. Then it
becomes a lot easier to approach our partners in a loving,
non-blaming manner.

Leila's Dream

*"It's the middle of the night and I hear noise
coming from the basement. I'm worried about the
baby in the nursery. I run downstairs and the
door to the basement is wide open and I see these
bear-like animals chained to the wall pulling at
the chain and growling. I run back up and into
the nursery and grab the baby from the crib and
scream for my husband."*

Read the dream again, and see every person, or animal or object in the dream as an expression of you. Ask yourself what are the characteristics of that object and why are they being called to your attention at this point. The dream might be letting you know that that character trait is part of you and you need to own it. You may want to experiment with "sensing" what it would feel like to become that person or animal. How would you move? What would you sound like?

"My parents used to always tell me that I had a terrible temper. I completely forgot about that until I went over the dream and saw those chained bears. I don't raise my voice with people. Even when I'm angry I try to play it down. But when I close my eyes during Body Truth and 'feel' the bear in me, I start making sounds I didn't even know I was capable of making. I've got a bunch of growling grizzlies in there and they're rattling their chains so hard, they're just about ready to bring the wall down. I've been keeping them chained up; I was too scared they'd end up hurting someone. Babies are so tiny, so vulnerable. What if I lost control and did something I'd regret? After a while the grizzlies turned out to be a lot less scary than I expected. One day they stretched out their paws the way dogs do and wanted to romp with me."

Jill's Dream

*"I'm in a park that has a garden café. My father
is sitting in the corner. I kiss him many times, I'm
so happy to see him. He is not alive or dead; he is
just there. It took a lot of effort for him to come.
He's tired. He came to say goodbye. I notice that
I'm not upset.
I walk out of the café and little monkeys take my
hand and lead me home."*

Understand that each dream is an invitation to change
something in your waking life, an attitude, belief, or behavior. What are you being asked to change this time?

"Our assignment in one of the phone circles was to get
a favorite children's book and read it to someone we love. I
knew exactly what book I wanted to read: Attic of the Wind
by Doris Herold Lund. My aunt gave it to me and my sister
when we were children. I asked my mom to send it to me,
and I read it to my husband a few days before this dream
came. It's about the Attic of the Wind, where all the things
you thought you lost are still floating around. My father
died when I was a baby, and for the last few months I've
been thinking about how sorrow and loss have been the
central themes of my life. In this dream I was not sad. My
father was tired, but he wasn't sad either. And he was not
alive but he wasn't dead. I can have a relationship with him
and it doesn't have to be sad.

"I've been thinking that the message of this lovely
worn old book, and the message of the dream – this image
of things not lost but swirling around you, beautiful, in the
sky – is part of the gift this baby is bringing to me."

Lucy's Dream

"I am in a long line with back-and-forth sections,
like at an airport. I am with my mom and sister.
Someone is very sick and going to die – we are all
in a line for assisted suicide, where we will lie
down at the end of the line and breathe in poison
and be carried onto the conveyor belt and then
be cremated. As we get closer to the end I start
to wonder why we are doing this – it suddenly
seems unnecessary to me. I pull my mom and sis-
ter out of the line and say, 'Why, are we doing
this? I don't want to. I know it might be hard but
I want to smell the roses.' And I get them both to
come with me; we get back in the car and we are
driving away."

Is the dream validating or rejecting a choice I've made in my waking life?

"My mom and my sister are prone to depression, and I've been pulled into the darkness much of my life. It feels like I've been just standing on this conveyor belt, not really moving myself, just being carried by habit, going through the same old stuff back and forth, over and over again. And now I'm starting to ask 'Why?' So it's wonderful to get this nod from God, and see that some very deep part of me is feeling strong enough to 'get back in the car,' and drive away, and leave all that behind. I went out this morning and bought a large bouquet of roses."

Lucy's dream is a most fitting way to conclude this part of the practice section. The image of choosing to "pull" ourselves and our loved ones out of the line that leads to destruction and a habitual, unexamined life is a perfect metaphor for the Fertile Heart work.

Chapter 15

Fertile Heart™ Body Truth

"I couldn't believe how much "NO" was in my feet when I asked myself if I was ready for this next baby. They started stomping and it looked like they'd never stop. I'm exhausted; time to really get off the infertility Mack truck and let time take its own path for a while before we start again. "

– Fertile Heart workshop participant

Once at a rehearsal of Romeo and Juliet, my scene partner, a strapping young actor, slapped his hand on my shoulder with such force my knees gave way and I almost toppled off the stage. I might've remained permanently lopsided if not for the massive shoulder pads that were in vogue in those days.

"No, no, no, Romeo!" The director's voice boomed from the back row. "She's not your drinking buddy! You have to show us how you feel about Juliet through the way you treat her: the way you tenderly take her hand, the way you follow her with your eyes when you part."

Your body wants the same thing. "No, no, no! Don't talk to me about love," it says. "Show me that you care through your behavior."

The practice of Body Truth is our chance to do just that: show the body that we care, that we want to hear what it has to say by giving it our undivided attention. It is a way we can give power and time to the intelligence that resides in the skin of the scalp, the heart muscle, the uterine wall, and every cell we're made of. The more willingly we do this, the more willingly and clearly will that intelligence articulate its preference.

As we discussed in "Issues in Our Tissues," the exercises that follow are meant to help us physicalize and release feelings rather than store them in our tissues; to invite the presence of the inner Ultimate Mom who will simply hold us with her attention, and observe compassionately without flinching, without judging or interpreting. Body Truth assists our Inner Orphans in being seen and heard, and eliminates the need for them to ask for attention in undesirable ways.

In order to trust you, the body will want to know that you're someone who'll make a date and keep it. Consistently. If you show up once in a while, and when you do, are less than fully attentive, not much will happen.

You'll need comfortable, loose clothing, a notebook, a designated Body Truth blanket, and a peaceful, private space. You may want to tell the other members of your household not to be alarmed if they hear you moan, groan, or make unusual utterances during your practice. The idea is to be as free in your expression as possible.

Getting your body moving, whether it's through a brisk walk, belly dancing, yoga, Gi Gong, or a boxing class, can be eminently useful, and I wholeheartedly invite you to seek out teachers of the modalities that appeal to you most. At the same time, the increased level of intimacy, insight, self-loving kindness, and freedom that comes from permitting the body to dictate its own movements and develop its own language is specific to Body Truth practice.

What follows are a series of guided movement sequences to get you started. A word of caution: this is not a competition, or an endurance test. Above all, be gentle with yourself, do not push the body beyond it's limits.

The Fertile Heart Body Truth CD offers a further in-depth exploration of this practice with additional movement sequences and a guided meditation titled, Riding the Current of Creation.

Follow the Longing

Intention:

To fully feel your desire and allow it to energize you.

Lie on your back with arms at your side, feet slightly apart. Close your eyes, bring your attention inward and follow the path of the breath for a few seconds. Invite an image of the life you long for. Draw the image into the body and let the longing move through you. Stretch your arms vertically over your head and reach. Pour all your longing into your outstretched arms, staying aware of the breath. Feel your entire upper body engaged in the stretch. Reach through the arms and the fingertips, as far as your longing takes you.

Breathe.

Release, and bring your arms back into neutral position alongside your body

Follow the path of the breath for a few seconds.

Stretch your arms over your head again, only this time include your lower body, your thigh muscles, all the way down to your toes.

Hold the stretch for a few seconds. Let the muscles speak the longing and continue to be aware of the breath. Release. If a sound wants to come through, open your mouth and let it out.

Breathe.

Release.

With your next inhalation gather into the palms of your hands all of your desire for a child, and make fists.

Breathe.

Tighten your fists and hold for a few seconds.

Breathe.

Release.

Open your mouth wide and allow sound to move through you.

Release, bring your arms back into neutral position alongside your body, and open your eyes.

If My Neck, Arm, Belly...Could Only Talk

Intention:
To identify feelings and ground yourself.

Lie down, arms at your side, feet slightly apart. Close your eyes, bring your attention inward and follow the path of the breath for a few seconds.

Scan your body and allow yourself to receive whatever feeling is present for you at this moment. On the scale of 1 to 10 let it be a 100. Is there a place in your body where you experience this feeling most distinctly?

Let the breath move through you.

With the next inhalation direct the breath toward the area where the feeling is most acute.

Breathe out through the mouth.

Let the breath move through you and ask: How would I move to articulate this feeling? Take your time, and bring awareness to each movement. Give your neck, your arms, your belly, your knees permission to speak their piece.

Don't censor; no one but you is listening.

When you feel complete, release, lie on your back with your arms alongside your body, and open your eyes.

The Wailing Wall

Intention:

To feel the support of something stronger than yourself.

When your body is filled with anguish or rage or any other difficult emotion, the Wailing Wall can be a lifesaver. My clients tell me they never realized what a supportive, non judgmental friend a wall can be.

Find an open space alongside the wall without any wall hangings, pictures, or furniture within five feet of where you are standing. Stand about a foot from the wall, facing it. Close your eyes, bring your attention inward and follow the path of the breath for a few seconds.

Lean forward with your palms firmly planted at about shoulder length on the section of wall in front of you. Allow yourself to feel any feelings that rise up in you at this moment.

Breathe.

Leaning against the wall, lift the right leg and shake it out, then do the same with the left leg. If your legs want to kick, let them, as long as you do so with awareness and are careful not to hurt yourself.

Breathe.

Bring your feet closer to the wall and stretch your arms above you. Let your fingers climb higher and higher up the wall, allowing yourself to fully experience the feeling coursing through you. If the feeling lifts you to your toes, let it.

Breathe and reach all the way through your fingertips.

If a sound comes, open your mouth and let it come fully.

When you feel complete, bring your arms down, release, and open your eyes.

.

Rock the Baby:

Intention:

To comfort and calm the body-child.

Lie on your back, close your eyes, bring your attention inward and follow the path of the breath for a few seconds.

Bring up your knees as far as you can without straining, and wrap your arms around them. Begin to gently rock in whatever rhythm feels most soothing. Give yourself permission to feel anything that comes up for you.

Open your chest, release your shoulders, and allow the breath to move through you freely.

Turn on your belly and bring your knees up and move rhythmically in an up and down motion, or side to side, whichever movement is more comforting.

When you feel complete, release, lie on your back with your arms alongside your body, and open your eyes.

Say No! Say Yes!

Intention:

To give yourself permission to wholeheartedly reject or embrace an idea and resolve inner conflicts.

You can do this sequence lying down or standing. Close your eyes, bring your attention inward and follow the path of the breath for a few seconds.

Invite an image of the conflict you're wrestling with. What is the response that rises up in your body at this moment? Is it a yes, or a no?

Choose one and ask various parts of your body to declare it as fully as possible.

How do your facial muscles say no? Do you shut your eyes and stick out your tongue? Do you grimace? How about the shoulders? Do they lift toward your ears, or tighten in resentment? Go through as many parts of your body as you wish.

When you feel complete, release, return to a neutral position lying on your back or standing with your arms alongside your body, and open your eyes.

To give yourself the opportunity to experience the opposite reaction, repeat the sequence of movements, allowing various body parts to declare "yes" as exuberantly as possible.

The Orphans

Intention:

To encourage the orphans inside you that are wrestling with jealousy, anger, disappointment, or other inconvenient emotions to speak their piece.

You can do this sequence lying down or standing. Close your eyes, bring your attention inward and follow the path of the breath for a few seconds.

Find a place in your body where you feel the feeling most intensely. How would your body speak this feeling through movement?

Breathe.

Listen inwardly for the voice of this orphan. What sound would best articulate her feelings?

Let the breath move through you and receive the presence of this orphaned part of you with unconditional compassion and kindness.

When you feel complete, release, return to a neutral position ~~lying on your~~ back or standing with your arms along-side your body, and open your eyes.

Child's Play

Intention:

To enliven and stimulate the body and the imagination and to add a little fun to your day. (To paraphrase an oft-repeated adage: We don't stop playing because we grow old, we grow old because we stop playing.)

Throughout the day, whether you're alone doing chores or in any other situation that allows for it, experiment with exaggerating your movements in a childlike manner. Skip, move your arms, walk around taking giant steps, throw punches at an invisible opponent, dance, or imitate the movement of an animal that has shown up in a dream. The idea is to increase the current of life force moving through you.

Go to the playground (even if it's difficult for you to watch so many *other people's* children; it's bound to be healing) and observe the bodies of small children. There is a rambunctious child within you that wants to move and play the way they do.

Flowing Fire

Intention:

To open ourselves to receive pleasure; to own and express sexual energy.

Stand with your feet shoulder width apart and your arms at your side. Close your eyes, bring your attention inward and follow the path of the breath for a few seconds.

Inhale through your nose and exhale through your

mouth, and gradually establish an invigorating rhythm of breathing.

When you're ready, swing your arms to accompany the breath.

With the next breath begin to bend and straighten your knees in the established rhythm. (Be careful not to lock the knees.)

Experiment with alternating between deeper and more shallow knee bends, and with a faster or slower rhythm. Bring your awareness into the genital area, and feel the energy of the movement flow and gather in your sexual organs.

Breathe out and return to a neutral position with arms at your side.

With the next breath rotate your hips in a rhythmic motion, inviting your torso and entire upper body to join in the undulating movement.

Breathe.

Return to a neutral position with arms at your side.

Lie down on your blanket, and let the breath move through you.

Close your eyes and invite a movement that's pleasurable and can be repeated at a steady rhythm. Ask your body to choose a rhythm and stay with it as long as you wish.

When you feel complete, release, return to a neutral position lying on your back with your arms alongside your body, and open your eyes.

Let It Be

Intention:
To make room for the body's innate intelligence to show you the way.

Start from a neutral position, lying on your back or standing up with your feet shoulder width apart, arms at your side.

Close your eyes, turn your attention inward, and follow the path of the breath for a few seconds.

Give your body unconditional permission to follow its own impulse, to move in a particular way or to remain unmoving.

Allow images, and thoughts to come and go and keep bringing your attention back to the breath.

Notice which movements inspire a change in your feelings.

When you feel that your body has said all it needed to say at this time, return to a neutral position lying on your back with your arms alongside your body, and open your eyes.

As with imagery, scan the movement sequences and choose one that feels the most liberating, challenging, or fun, and begin. You can also refer to the *Fertile Heart Body Truth* CD for a guided Body Truth meditation and for additional sequences.

Consistent practice will enlarge your vocabulary of movement, allow you to hear your body's call for attention more clearly, and make you feel more connected to yourself and others. For us humans, life was meant to be primarily an "in the body" experience.

Chapter 16

Feeding the Body-Child

"For the first two days of my cycle the pain used to be so bad, even with a painkiller, that I had to stay in bed. Since I've cut out all wheat, sugar, soy and almost all diary and meat, this is the second month I've been able to stop painkillers and actually go to work. I still feel some cramping, but it's nothing in comparison.".

– Fertile Heart workshop participant

In this section you'll find a brief list of foods and a handful of recipes that illustrate the ideas I talked about in the "Ally in the Cupboard" chapter. You may want to reread it to remind yourself of the potential havoc caused by foes, and the good that comes from choosing to eat well. Included are suggestions to help you cleanse the digestive system, lighten its workload, encourage hormonal balance, tilt your body ecology toward a more alkaline environment, and provide a variety of fertility-boosting nutrients.

The resident chef in our home and the consultant for the Cooking Corner of our website, www.fertileheart.com, is my husband, Edward Baum, a graduate of the Culinary Institute of America. Before he became a computer programmer, Ed worked for ten years as a professional chef. His creativity in the kitchen is what made my transition from junk food addict to health enthusiast such a tasty adventure.

When you first decide to experiment with food as a tool, you might want to take a field trip to a health food store or a supermarket that carries organic produce and a variety of items with healthful ingredients. It's a good idea to eat before your field trip (otherwise you won't have the patience to do what's needed) and to give yourself lots of time to explore, read labels, and taste at the deli counter. You might want to make your own list ahead of time, of "friend foods" to try.

To review, here is a list of items and ingredients to avoid, and a list of beneficial ones. Neither of these is an exhaustive inventory, but simply a guide to get you started. Remember to experiment! No matter how healthy the food, when we eat the same flavor and ingredients every day, we can overstimulate particular organs and cause harm. For example, eating too much seaweed can overstimulate the thyroid and throw off hormonal balance. The more varied the ingredients and combinations on your plate, and the more colorful, the more likely you'll receive the nutrients you need.

"No" Foods and Ingredients

Alcohol – weakens immune system; acid-forming; interferes with mineral absorption, causing nutrient deficiency; can impair ovulation by raising prolactin levels. (Prolactin is a hormone that stimulates the production of breast milk and inhibits ovulation.

Caffeine – interferes with the liver's processing of excess estrogen, disrupting hormonal balance. (Estrogen is one of the key fertility hormones.) Caffeine also weakens the nervous system and immune function; can cause calcium depletion.

Processed soy (soy cheeses and myriad of products containing soy, including tofu and soy milk) – linked with loss of libido, impaired mineral absorption, and disruption of thyroid function, (See exceptions and further discussion in the "Yes" Foods and Ingredients column!)

Dairy – If your health history and constitution indicate congestion, fibroids, cysts, or endometriosis, you may want to exclude all dairy products from your meals. They are mucus-producing; in some people milk consumption might be linked to fibroid and cyst formation, as well as endometriosis. Excess calcium also taxes the kidneys, the organs responsible for regulating the acid-alkaline balance in the blood.

White flour – raises blood insulin levels; disrupts endocrine function; weakens immune system; is implicated in a long list of chronic, degenerative diseases.

Processed sugar – can increase acidity; causes mineral deficiencies; weakens immune function. If sugar is difficult to omit, you may want to experiment with a small amount of treats made with natural sweeteners and eat them slowly and mindfully. A craving for sugar might indicate magnesium deficiency. Be sure to include dark leafy vegetables, whole grains, and beans in your meals to correct this possible imbalance.

Highly processed vegetable and seed oils – cottonseed oil, safflower, sunflower, and corn oil, among others (see discussion in "Ally in the Cupboard").

Canola oil – There is much controversy around canola oil, I choose not to use it because it goes rancid easily and there are several studies that indicate a possible harmful effect on cardiovascular health.

Peanuts – Although the peanut has a number of healthful properties, it is a highly allergenic food, susceptible to the growth of aflatoxin, a known carcinogen. If you choose to eat peanut butter, you may want to grind it yourself. Avoid products containing hydrogenated stabilizing oils.

Peas – contain m-xylohydroquinone, a natural contraceptive.

Ginger - Avoid it if you're pregnant; otherwise ginger is a cleansing and warming food that enhances circulation.

"Yes" Foods and Ingredients

All the items below should be organic whenever possible.

Vegetables

Dark leafy greens – good source of folic acid, calcium, vitamin A and C, B vitamins, and a number of minerals.

Spinach – must be blanched or lightly cooked to deactivate the effect of oxalic acid, which removes iron and calcium from the body. Good source of vitamin B6, which helps maintain estrogen-progesterone balance; B1, B2, E, carotenes, iron, magnesium, and manganese. (Progesterone is a hormone necessary for maintaining a healthy pregnancy.)

Chard – many different varieties of chard are available, all highly nutritious. Chard belongs to the same family as spinach and must also be blanched or lightly cooked to deactivate the effect of oxalic acid. It's a good source of chlorophyll, vitamin C, calcium, niacin, folic acid, fiber, and zinc, a mineral which is essential for healthy male sex hormone function, protein synthesis and cell growth, as well as immune function.

Kale – good source of calcium, iron, beta-carotene, and folic acid. Kale, broccoli, cauliflower, and cabbage contain goitrogens, compounds that interfere with the production of thyroid hormones. Cooking helps deactivate the goitrogenic effect, so if you suspect hypothyroidism, you're best to avoid eating these foods raw. If you're eating a significant amount of kale and other cruciferous vegetables, be sure to also consume an adequate amount of iodine-rich foods, such as sea vegetables.

Lettuce – the darker the color, the richer the nutrient content. Romaine lettuce is a good source of chlorophyll, vitamin K, B1, B2, chromium, and manganese. Iceberg lettuce is a good source of choline. Since choline is an essential nutrient required for proper metabolism of fats, it plays an important role in healthy hormone function. (Estrogen is both produced and stored in our fat cells.)

Daikon – All vegetables in the radish family have hormone-balancing properties, but daikon is the one most favored for its medicinal effect. It contains a group of sulfur-based chemicals that support the flow of bile, enhancing liver and gallbladder function.

Avocado – good source of healthful monounsaturated fatty acids, B vitamins, vitamin E, and potassium.

Wheatgrass – juiced, a good source of chlorophyll, folic acid, and a number of minerals.

After the publication of *Inconceivable*, people who misunderstood the role of wheatgrass in my self-healing regimen began to perpetuate a myth of wheatgrass being a remedy for lowering follicle-stimulating-hormone (FSH) levels. Wheatgrass is a powerful blood cleanser and antioxidant, but drinking wheatgrass was no more than one tiny piece of my story. As far as I know, there is no direct link between wheatgrass consumption and FSH levels.

Celery – great source of folic acid, B6 and B1, and potassium – important nutrients for enhancing endocrine function.

Cucumber – contains folic acid, vitamins A and C, and potassium, magnesium, and other minerals.

Carrot – great source of carotenes, antioxidant compounds, vitamin K, biotin, vitamin C, B6, and minerals.

Beet – Beet greens and roots are a good source of B6, iron, magnesium, and phosphorus, and serve as excellent detoxifying agents as they enhance liver and bowel function.

Shiitake mushrooms – a high-protein vegetable with immune-enhancing properties, plus a good source of selenium. (Avoid if you suspect endometriosis or yeast infections.)

Garlic, onions, raw and cooked – sources of magnesium, vitamin B6, selenium (to strengthen immune function.) Researchers at Pennsylvania State University found that crushing garlic and letting it sit for 10 minutes helps preserve more of its healthful properties. To get the maximum benefit, eat garlic raw or cooked lightly.

Fruits – preferably in season

Green apple –lowest sugar content of all varieties. Apples in general are a good source of pectin, a soluble fiber that enhances bowel function.

Grapes – good source of flavonoids, vitamin B6, thiamine, riboflavin, vitamin C, potassium.

Cherries – excellent source of flavonoids, vitamin C, and copper.

Apricots – good source of immune-enhancing carotenes.

Blueberries – superb source of antioxidants; strengthens the digestive system.

Tibetan Goji berries – hailed in Asian medicine as a libido enhancer; excellent source of amino acids, and trace minerals.

Grapefruits, oranges – rind rich in antioxidants and bioflavonoids, which promote the formation of a healthy uterine lining.

Lemons – contain vitamin C, flavonoids, and potassium.

Whole Grains

Quinoa – a high-protein grain, it contains essential amino acids important for tissue formation.

Millet – a good source of B vitamins; has been touted in macrobiotic literature as a hormone balancer. Note that millet contains a goitrogen, so be sure to alternate with other grains.

Brown rice – good source of fiber, essential amino acids, and B vitamins, including B6. Experiment with the many varieties of brown rice available.

Amaranth – high-protein content, B vitamins, calcium, potassium, manganese, and copper, a source of phytosterols, compounds that show promise in preventing degenerative diseases.

Fermented Soy Products

In the last decade there has been much controversy about the health-enhancing properties of soy. The current consensus points toward fermented soy's being the only health-enhancing form of this food. As I pointed out earlier in this chapter, non fermented soy has been linked with loss of libido, impaired mineral absorption, and disruption of thyroid function. From reports of clients who've suffered from endometriosis and fibroids, avoiding all foods with estrogenic effect has been most helpful in reducing symptoms.

Avoid fermented foods as well as bread products made with yeast if you are prone to yeast infections. Consumption of fermented soy products can be particularly useful to women who have estrogen deficiencies.

Miso – a fermented soybean paste, miso has been a mainstay of Japanese cooking for hundreds of years. It is a source of valuable healing enzymes, helps build up our blood, aids digestion, and is particularly useful in the assimilation of carbohydrates. There are many varieties of miso, ranging from white, lightly aged barley miso to dark brown soy miso. Generally, the more it is aged the darker the color and stronger the flavor. It might be good to start with a milder variety and work your way up to the hard stuff. Because enzymes are destroyed by heating food above 118 degrees F, and some of their power is lost above 105 degrees F, miso should always be added after all other ingredients have achieved their desired consistency.

Tempeh – cakes of fermented soybeans, they're a good source of protein, B vitamins, copper, iron, and manganese.

Tamari – soy sauce made by fermenting soybeans with mold. I prefer to use the low-sodium brand.

Beans

Beans are an excellent source of fiber, which makes them useful in improving blood sugar levels. They combine with grains into complete proteins, and are good sources of B vitamins, folic acid, and trace minerals necessary for production of enzymes. One such enzyme, sulfite oxidase, enhances aspects of liver function. Since the liver is one of the key estrogen-processing organs, this might be one of the reasons why some sources cite beans as a fertility enhancing food. The easiest to digest are adzuki beans; red kidney beans are high in antioxidants. The added bonus is that beans and lentils are associated with reduced risk of breast cancer. Soaking beans before cooking makes them easier to digest.

Sea Vegetables

Hijiki – a stringy, rich-tasting sea vegetable, it's a wonderful source of iodine, calcium, iron, and minerals.

Arame – a milder tasting variety of seaweed.

Kombu – a thick variety of sea vegetable that increases the mineral content of soups, grain, and bean dishes. Might have a mild laxative effect.

Agar-agar – a gelatin-like substance made from several species of seaweeds, and used in Japanese tradition for hundreds of years. It comes in bars or flakes, is a good source of calcium, iron, and trace minerals, and is said to reduce inflammation and carry toxic and radioactive waste out of the body. Some holistic practitioners recommend eating foods made with agar-agar during and after air travel. Note: Agar-agar has a mild laxative effect.

Nuts, Nut Butters, and Seeds

Nuts, nut butters, and seeds are excellent sources of key vitamins and minerals, as well as healthy fat, which is essential for hormone production. Be sure to refrigerate all nuts to avoid rancidity; it's best to purchase these foods in stores that have a high volume and quick turnover. Unprocessed, raw, unsalted nuts are most healthful.

Almonds – Soaking raw almonds for eight to twelve hours makes them easier to digest. They're a good source of vitamin E, monounsaturated and polyunsaturated oils, flavonoids, potassium, zinc, and calcium, and an excellent source of boron.

Cashews – contain minerals, copper, magnesium, potassium, iron, zinc, biotin, and protein.

Sunflower seeds – good source of vitamin E.

Pumpkin seeds – magnesium, phosphorus, iron, zinc, copper, B1, B2, B3, and protein.

Sesame seeds – Hulled sesame seeds are a great source of protein, calcium, antioxidants, vitamins B1, B2, and zinc, Tahini is a delicious sesame seed paste.

Brazil nuts – excellent source of selenium, zinc.

Oils

Note: Avoid hydrogenated and low-fat products, which have been stripped of beneficial fat.

Olive oil – cold-pressed, extra virgin olive oil has the

highest level of healthful oleic acid, an omega 9-monoun-saturated fatty acid. While olive oil is the healthiest fat you can use, it can contribute to the buildup of body fat, so do not overuse.

Coconut oil – contains lauric acid, a health-promoting fat with antibacterial properties.

Sesame oil – Restrict use to a small amount, used as a flavoring agent; its high content of omega 6 fatty acids can contribute to impaired immune and endocrine function.

Sweeteners

Use sweeteners sparingly.

Honey – B6, B2, and iron. Benefits vary depending on processing.

Black strap molasses – contains iron, calcium, potassium, magnesium, and selenium.

Brown rice syrup – a complex sugar (polysaccharide). This is a translucent, mild-flavored sweetener that does not cause a rapid rise in blood sugar levels.

Fish

Check fish advisories in your area. (The following link provides national and local consumption advisories: http://epa.gov/waterscience/fish/.)

If you choose to eat other animal food, look for hormone, antibiotic, and cruelty-free sources.

Supplements and
Additional Endocrine Boosters

Although the synergy of nutrients in naturally occurring foods cannot be replicated in any lab, and supplements alone will not correct an underlying imbalance, some supplementation might be useful. Depending on your particular hormonal and physical profile, you may want to explore the benefits of some of the following:

A multivitamin/mineral – food-based brands are more easily assimilated. I like to divide the dosage, and take it at two different times during the day.

B-complex – essential for a healthy nervous system, and especially important if you're following a vegetarian diet

Folic acid - plays a key role in cell division and fetal development.

Boron - a trace mineral which helps the body utilize estrogen. Women with low estrogen levels or elevated FSH levels might consider taking a low-dose boron supplement. In one study, 3 milligrams of boron per day increased estrogen levels in postmenopausal women. In the same study, boron proved to have a positive effect on calcium absorption, thus reducing the risk of osteoporosis.

Omega 3 oil (fish oil) – regulates hormone synthesis, supports healthy cervical mucus, and acts as an anti-inflammatory agent. Note: Because of its blood -thinning properties, people who are taking anticoagulant drugs should avoid fish oil supplements.

Royal jelly (discontinue if you're pregnant) – energizing, and has been used in a number of healing traditions as a natural remedy for strengthening the male and female reproductive systems. You may want to test for allergic reactions by ingesting a very small amount of this nutrient at first.

Green tea (decaffeinated) – contains catechins, a powerful antioxidant with fertility enhancing and rejuvenating properties

Pycnogenol – a potent antioxidant. Studies indicate that it is effective in enhancing sperm quality.

Co-enzyme Q-10 – is reported to improve the utilization of oxygen on a cellular level, and is thus useful in tissue repair.

Chlorella - the most gently cleansing of the microalgae, detoxifying by binding with heavy metals; highly nutritional; regulates cellular repair.

Probiotic – supports digestion by replenishing the beneficial bacteria in the gastrointestinal tract.

Milk thistle – an excellent, gentle liver tonic; use during the cleansing phase of your healing process, then discontinue.

L-arginine – An amino acid, it is said to enhance the secretion of growth hormones by the pituitary gland, and to relax the blood vessels, thus increasing blood flow. L-arginine, unlike other supplements, should be taken on an empty stomach. Note: The herpes virus utilizes L-arginine; therefore, supplementation may reactivate an existing herpes virus.

There is much enthusiasm in both the allopathic and holistic world about L-arginine and DHEA, a growth hormone. But any responsible caregiver will agree that supplements that tamper with growth hormones should be approached with caution, and discontinued after a reasonable time period.

With supplements, as with any other medicinal remedies, it's best to introduce one compound at a time and CAREFULLY OBSERVE your body's response. Take dosages as recommended on the product label or consult with a health care provider knowledgeable in the area of supplementation and natural remedies.

Before we move on to the recipes, here are some commonsense health-and fertility-enhancing habits that I, and just about everyone I know, needs to be reminded of from time to time.

One of the necessities, and great joys of parenting is the ability to feed our children well. This may sound radical, but the way I see it, it's unlikely that you can be a good parent to yourself or to your child without knowing how to prepare a nourishing, healthy meal. So, dive into the adventure of cooking. To paraphrase Franklin Roosevelt, there is nothing to fear but fear itself, or in my case, a few burned pots and inedible concoctions. But the confidence that comes with learning how to feed yourself and your family is worth the effort.

If you're having an intense emotional reaction to something or someone, use a Body Truth sequence, or imagery exercise to release it as much as you can before sitting down to eat. Otherwise you'll be eating your rage along with your salad, and adding a difficult-to-digest ingredient to your meal.

Before you begin eating, follow your breath until you feel centered, and invite a sense of gratitude for the nourishment you're about to receive.

Digestion begins in the mouth. Chewing slowly and with attention, and doing your best to coat your food in saliva, fosters patience and is essential for lightening the work of the digestive system. You might find it easier to concentrate on chewing if you put down your utensils after each mouthful.

Eating your meals at the same time each day sends a message to your body–child that you are reliable. The more your body learns to trust and unclench, the more willingly it allows the life force to flow through you.

During mealtimes, choose to be fully present to the experience of feeding yourself. Eat your meals sitting down without doing anything else. If that's too much to ask for, calming, pleasurable reading might be a good choice of activity until you can learn to focus entirely on "feeding the body-child."

Allow at least fifteen to twenty minutes for meals. If at all possible, aim to make lunch your largest meal. If that's too much of a challenge, eat your evening meal about three hours before bedtime. Your stomach needs to be as empty as possible to allow your body to repair, cleanse, and balance itself during the night.

Estrogen is both produced and stored in your fat cells. Levels of body fat can therefore significantly hinder or increase your chances of pregnancy. I have found that many of my students have gradually balanced their weight, not by focusing on weight loss or gain, but by simply changing their relationship to food.

Foods high in fiber, such as grains and vegetables, are necessary for elimination of excess estrogen and other waste material. This in turn supports hormonal balance, as well as the proper functioning of all vital organs. Adequate fiber is also useful in lightening the workload of the liver, the organ responsible for processing estrogen.

Foods that have a laxative effect (cause contractions) should be used sparingly or not at all after you become pregnant.

If your constitution allows it, include some raw or fermented, enzyme-rich foods with every meal. Food enzymes are essential for proper digestion and absorption of nutrients. They are de-activated by cooking. When we eat an overabundance of cooked food, our pancreas is called upon to compensate for a lack of digestive enzymes. Miso, olive oil, and avocados are good sources of food enzymes.

It is best not to drink for at least a half hour to forty-five minutes before and after meals. Liquids dilute the digestive juices and secretions and result in impaired assimilation of nutrients.

Experiment and see what works best with your temperament and constitution.

With food as with everything else, common sense and moderation can go a long way. Just because a certain food can help balance hormones doesn't mean that excessive quantities of it will balance your hormones more efficiently.

To stimulate your lymphatic system (plays a key role in immune function) brush your skin daily with a soft bristle brush. Before showering, brush with light rapid strokes toward your heart starting at your feet and moving on to your arms and upper body. Gentle bouncing on a mini trampoline can also energize the lymph system.

One of the most effective activities to stimulate the immune system, balance hormones, and allow the self-regulating mechanism of the body to do its job is fasting. Observe a daily mini-fast. If you put at least twelve hours between dinner and breakfast, your breakfast will be what it has always been meant to be: a breaking of the fast. Many people find a twenty-four-hour vegetable juice or broth fast once a week or once every two weeks to be highly beneficial, especially in the first few months of your Fertile Heart practice

If we wish to maximize the healing properties of food, steadfastness is the key, rather than waves of enthusiasm followed by apathy. If you find yourself regressing to old habits, chances are the Inner Orphans are asking for attention. This is the time to kindly and patiently take yourself by the hand and begin again. (Imagery, Body Talk, and dream work can be useful.)

Our task, then, is to use food to cleanse, nourish, and fortify us; to ease digestion; to alkalize our bodies, and to delight the senses, the heart, and the soul.

Recipes

The recipes that follow are meant to be departure points for your own culinary adventures.

Morning Cleansing Suggestions

Green Lemonade Cleansing Cocktail

I find that many of my clients tend to make their juices much too sweet when they first begin juicing. Since the relationship between high levels of blood sugar and ovarian function has been clearly established, it makes sense to reduce the amount of sweetening agents in all your prepared food.

Ingredients:
  1 peeled lemon
  2 celery stalks
  6 or more dark green lettuce leaves
  ½ cucumber with skin
  1 green apple

Directions:
  Blend all ingredients in juicer and sip slowly.

In the macrobiotic tradition celery and carrot are considered helpful with ovulation irregularities. You may want to replace the cucumber with a medium- sized- carrot two or three times a week. In cold weather I like to heat up my juice slightly and drink it warm.

Serves one.

Carrot Salad Liver Tonic

The liver is responsible for processing excess estrogen and other toxins, which is no easy task. This salad is a great way to show your support for this often overworked and underloved organ. One of my nutritionist friends recommends eating this carrot salad every morning for seven days as a liver cleanser.

Ingredients:
   3 medium size shredded carrots
   1 tablespoon of cold - pressed organic olive oil
   Juice of 1 lemon

Combine and eat.
Serves one.

Balancing Daikon Broth

To maximize the medicinal properties of this broth, it is suggested that you drink it every other day for three weeks and observe your body's response. You can create a useful variation of this broth by adding one medium-sized carrot.

Ingredients:
   1 medium daikon sliced
   1 strip kombu rinsed (approximately 3 inch piece)
   1 ½ cups water

Directions:
   Place ingredients into a pot and bring to a boil.
   Turn down the heat and simmer covered for twenty minutes.
   Drink broth warm.

Serves one.

Miso from Mana

This recipe comes from Lee at 'Mana', one of my favorite restaurants in New York.

Ingredients:
>   1 strip kombu rinsed (approximately 3 inch piece)
>   4 cups water
>   3 tablespoons white mellow miso paste
>   1 teaspoon tamari

Directions:
>   Bring water with kombu to a boil. Then simmer for 3 minutes.
>   Remove kombu.
>   Remove from heat and pour about ½ cup of the broth into a separate small bowl. Add miso into the bowl and mix until smooth.
>   Slowly stir the miso into the soup.
>   Add tamari and serve.

If you want to reheat the soup be careful not to boil, otherwise you will destroy the enzymes.

Variations include adding wakame, squash, carrots and/or shitake mushrooms after removing the kombu and before adding the miso, then simmering until the vegetables are the desired consistency.

Experiment with different varieties of Miso.

Try adding fresh chopped scallions right before serving.

Serves two to four.

Blood - Building Beet Salad

Beets are high in iron, and therefore are effective blood
builders. They're also cleansing- and digestion-promoting
agents.

Ingredients:
4 beets
1 teaspoon sesame oil
1 teaspoon honey

Directions:
Clean beets and place whole and unpeeled in a pot
with just enough water to cover.
Add honey and sesame oil to the water.
Bring to a boil, then simmer for 1½ - 2 hours or until
a knife easily inserts.
Cool beets, peel, slice and enjoy.
Serve cold or warm.

Serves two to four.

The "Spring Cleaning" chapter in *Inconceivable* might offer
added inspiration on cleansing.

Lunch Suggestions

Digesting protein-rich foods such as nuts, flesh foods (fish or chicken), or fermented soy such as tempeh takes energy and time. If you eat them before 3 P.M., your body will have enough time and energy to digest them and assimilate the nutrients. If you work outside the home, you may want to invest in a stainless steel thermos/food jar.

Tempeh Temptation

Since soy products tax your thyroid, be sure to combine soy with iodine-rich foods like seaweed, kelp, asparagus, and white onion to support your thyroid function.

Ingredients:
  1 (8-ounce) package tempeh
  1 teaspoon sesame oil
  1 tablespoon honey
  1 tablespoon tamari
  Juice of 1 lemon

Directions:
  Cut tempeh into approximately 1-inch wide by ¼-inch deep by 3-inch long strips.
  Combine all wet ingredients; (Add a little water if the mixture is too thick)
  Add tempeh and marinate for fifteen minutes.
  Lay out tempeh strips on baking dish
  Broil for three to five minutes, then flip and continue broiling for another 2-3 minutes
  Check often to make sure they don't burn.
  Serve with marinated greens, asparagus, or salad of your choice.

  Serves two to four.

Lecso a la Woodstock (pronounced lehcho)

This is a variation on one of my favorite childhood dishes, and I like it best served over short-grain brown rice.

Ingredients:
4 medium to large onions sliced, not diced (4 cups)
4 medium to large green peppers, sliced into thin strips
4 medium to large ripe tomatoes, or 2 cans of peeled tomatoes diced
2-4 teaspoon chopped garlic
1 tablespoon olive oil
¼ cup water
1 tablespoon sweet paprika
1- 3 tablespoons salt (season to taste)

Directions:
In a large pot heat olive oil and water. (The oil helps the assimilation of fat-soluble vitamins.)
Add onions.
Cook over medium heat, stirring frequently.
As the water evaporates and the onions start to brown, be careful to not let them stick and burn. If they start to stick, add a little more water.
Add the rest of the ingredients.
Bring to a boil, then lower heat and simmer approximately one hour.

Serves four to six.

You can add tempeh or another meat-like substance. This dish also works well with garbanzo beans.

Wonder Wraps

Ingredients:
>   Brown rice – cooked
>   Avocado – sliced
>   Lettuce – chopped
>   Cucumbers – sliced
>   Veggies – sliced
>   Fermented vegetables

You can make wraps with rice, beans, veggies, lettuce, humus, avocados, and just about anything else. It's fun to simply lay out a variety of ingredients on the table and have everyone make their own version of the Wonder Wrap. I like to use the packaged organic chapatis that they carry at my local health food store, but there are a lot of different products on the market.

Adi's Asparagus

Ingredients:
>   1 bunch asparagus
>   ¼ cup water
>   1 tablespoon olive oil
>   1 teaspoon chopped garlic
>   1 tablespoon tamari

Directions:
>   Heat pan with the water and oil.
>   Add garlic for one minute or until it starts to dry out.
>   Add the asparagus, stir to coat with garlic and oil.
>   Add a tablespoon of water and cook about two to four
>   minutes, stirring continually to make sure that the

asparagus doesn't burn.
Add tamari and a little water, keep stirring until
the asparagus is coated with the tamari and is dry.

The challenge here is to cook the asparagus long
enough that it's dry but not so long that it's over-
cooked.
Serve with a grain and/or tempeh.

Serves two to four.

Vegetable Sushi

Ingredients:

A package of nori (seaweed) sheets
A variety of raw vegetables
Brown rice (cooked; you can add a little soy sauce to
the cooking water to add flavor)
A small bowl of water

Directions:
Cut up all vegetables into small strips.
Take a sheet of nori, put an inch-wide layer of rice
at one end of the sheet, place the vegetable strips
over the rice, and roll up slowly, making sure the
roll is tight.
As you're about to close up the roll, wet your finger
slightly and smooth out the top of the nori sheet with
your wet finger. It will help the two ends of the sheet
to stick together.
Cut up into smaller sushi pieces

Dinner Suggestions

Hearty Vegetable Soup

Soups are easy to digest, and generally mineral-rich. Some of my clients who have had a history of repeated miscarriages discovered that their diet lacked mineral content, and have found this vegetable soup especially helpful in correcting that problem. Kale and chard should cook between twenty and thirty minutes.

Ingredients:
>3 medium to large onions, diced (3 cups)
>2-4 teaspoons garlic, chopped
>1 tablespoon olive oil
>3 large carrots, diced (2 cups)
>1 celery stalk, diced (½ cup)
>4 medium potatoes cut in large pieces (2 cups)
>½ head cauliflower, in small flowers (1 ½ cups)
>½ small bunch kale, cut into 1" squares (2 cups)
>½ small bunch chard, cut into 1" squares (2 cups)
>½ small head broccoli (1 ½ cups)
>Shiitake mushrooms thinly sliced (1 cup)
>8 - 10 cups water (enough to cover)
>1 teaspoon thyme
>1 teaspoon sweet paprika
>1 - 3 tablespoons salt (season to taste)

Directions:
>Into a large pot place onions, ½ the garlic, oil and ¼ cup of water.
>Cook on medium heat, stirring occasionally. Be careful to not let the onions stick and burn.
>Cook until the onions are translucent.
>Add mushrooms, carrots, celery, thyme, paprika and

4 cups of water.

Bring to a boil, then lower heat and simmer approximately twenty minutes.

Add potatoes, chard, kale and cauliflower, and water if necessary to cover, and simmer 20 - 25 minutes.

When the potatoes are tender, add the broccoli and remaining garlic and simmer three to five more minutes.

Season with salt and/or soy sauce to taste.

For extra calcium, herbalist Susun Weed recommends adding a couple of tablespoons of raw almond butter. Make sure your digestive tract is up for it.

Serves six to eight.

Adjust the quantities of the various ingredients to taste. Try different spices: rosemary, oregano, basil, bay leaves.

Lentil Soup

There are several types of lentils: brown, red, green, yellow. Many health food stores, specialty shops, and large groceries or supermarkets should have them available. Red are the smallest and cook more quickly. The green, or 'French' variety, are smaller, stay a little firmer, maintain their shape and are my favorite. The brown, which is the most common type in North America, are somewhere in the middle. You should experiment with different types. The cooking method is the same, but the cooking time and consistency will vary slightly.

Ingredients:
> 4 medium to large onions diced (4 cups)
> 2 medium carrots diced (1 ½ cups)
> 2-4 teaspoons chopped garlic
> 1 tablespoon olive oil
> 1 tablespoon sweet paprika
> 1 pound lentils
> 6 cups of water
> 1 - 2 tablespoons salt (season to taste)

Directions:
> Into a large pot place onions, garlic, oil and ¼ cup of water.
> Cook on medium heat, stirring occasionally. Be careful to not let the onions stick and burn.
> Cook until the onions are translucent.
> Wash the lentils and add to the onions and garlic. Add water.
> Bring to a boil, then lower heat and simmer approximately an hour and a half to two hours.
> Season with salt and/or soy sauce to taste. (Actually, I like to use salt during the cooking process and season to just under the desired taste, and then finish

with soy sauce when serving. It adds a nice touch.)

Serves six to eight.

Hijiki Joy Salad

Ingredients:
 4 tablespoons of black hijiki
 Juice of one small lemon
 Dash of sesame oil
 1 - 2 tablespoons of low - sodium tamari soy sauce
 1 carrot, cut into matchsticks
 ½ daikon, cut into matchsticks (½ - ¾ cup)
 1 teaspoon of grated fresh ginger

Directions:
 Wash hijiki, quickly, to retain nutrients.
 Place in a bowl and cover with water.
 Skim off any impurities that rise to the top, and continue to soak for five minutes.
 Drain the hijiki, but reserve some of the soaking water as for cooking.
 Place hijiki, carrots, and daikon, 1/2 cup with a dash of tamari in the skillet and sauté for three minutes.
 Add the rest of the water until it covers the hijiki and the vegetables and bring to a boil.
 Reduce heat and simmer for forty-five minutes.
 Add the rest of the tamari, sesame oil, and simmer for an additional ten minutes.
 Remove from heat, and add lemon and ginger.
 Mix and serve.

Combines beautifully with most vegetables, grains, or tempeh. I like it mixed with short grain brown rice.

Serves four.

Marinated Vegetable Medley

Ingredients:

    1 small head Romaine or Red Leaf lettuce
        (cut into 1-inch squares) (4 cups)
    1 large carrot, diced small
    1 large red pepper, diced small
    1 endive, diced small
    1 green pepper, diced small
    1 small summer squash or zucchini, diced small
    1 bunch of radishes, diced small
    1 tablespoon garlic, chopped
    ¼ cup lemon juice
    1 tablespoon tamari
    Dash of sesame oil

Directions:

    Place vegetables in a bowl.

    Mix garlic, lemon juice, tamari, and sesame oil.

    Pour marinade over vegetables and toss until all vegetables are coated.

    Marinate in the refrigerator from one to twenty-four hours before serving, occasionally retossing in the marinade. For added nutrients and fun, you can add pumpkin or sunflower seeds.

Serves four to six.

Spicy Pasta with Vegetables and Avocado

Ingredients:
  3 cups cooked organic brown rice pasta
  1 teaspoon sea salt
  ½ cup olive oil
  1 cup cucumbers diced
  1 cup green, red, and yellow peppers, diced
  1 avocado, sliced
  ½ teaspoon freshly ground black pepper
  1 teaspoon paprika
  1 teaspoon dried oregano
  ¼ - ½ teaspoon cayenne pepper

Directions:
  Pour olive oil over pasta and mix.
  Add vegetables and spices.
  Top with slices of avocado.

  You can make a cooked variation of this dish and steam- sauté the vegetables (except the avocado) first in a little bit of water until they reach the desired tenderness. When preparing pasta, adding enzyme-rich olive oil after cooking will make it easier to digest.

Serves four

Browned Millet with Onions

Millet is the fertility wonder grain, highly touted as a hormone balancer. There are a great many reasons for learning to love millet. It is the high - protein grain with an alkaline effect. It's very easy to digest, and combines beautifully with just about any food.

Ingredients:
    1 cup millet
    ½ cup onions, diced small
    ¼ teaspoon salt
    1 tablespoon olive oil
    4 cups boiling water

Directions:
    Place the millet in a pot or skillet over low - medium heat stirring frequently until brown.
    Remove the millet from the pot when it starts to give off a nutty aroma.
    Cook onions in water and oil until transparent.
    Add all ingredients together
    Cover tightly and simmer for thirty to forty minutes, or until all water is absorbed.

Serves two to four

Quinoa Salad

Ingredients:
>3 cups cooked quinoa
>¼ cup onions, chopped fine
>1 cup cucumbers, diced small
>¼ cup lemon juice
>½ cup olive oil
>1 tablespoon garlic, chopped fine
>½ teaspoon cumin
>Sea salt and other spices of your choice to taste
>Dill would be another option.

Directions:
>Toss all ingredients together lightly and refrigerate several hours to allow flavors to be absorbed

Serves four

Snacks and Treats

Just in case you need a quick reminder: Reducing your intake of sugar (I mean any kind of sugar, including the organic, wheat-free carob chip cookies in aisle four) will boost ovarian function and your immune system. As we discussed in the "Ally in the Cupboard" chapter, usually it's our heart, not our stomach, that craves sweets. So if curbing your sweet tooth is difficult for you, you may want to think about other ways to "be sweet on yourself." That said, with a little creativity you can come up with nutrient-filled treats that will even enhance your endocrine system. As you begin to wean yourself off sweets, experiment with reducing the amount of sweetening agents you use.

Ellena's Excellent Brown Rice Pudding

This is an easy recipe, but takes time, about four hours, to cook. It is, however, worth the wait. I like it best served warm.

Ingredients:
  1 cup short-grain brown rice
  1 ½ quarts rice milk
  ¼ cup brown rice syrup
  2 tablespoons vanilla
  ½ teaspoon salt

Directions:
  Wash rice.
  Combine all ingredients in a pot.
  Bring to a boil and then reduce flame to as low as possible.
  Stir every fifteen minutes. (It is important to watch this more closely as time goes by, as you increase the risk of cooking off the liquid and burning the rice.)
  If it gets dry, add some water. Top with cinnamon and serve warm or cold.

Prufrock's Peach Kanten

(Named after my favorite line from T.S. Eliot's poem "The Love Song of J. Alfred Prufrock," "Do I dare to eat a peach?") Kanten is a gelatin-like food.

Ingredients:
  2 ½ tablespoons agar flakes
  2 cups peach nectar

1 cups fruit, sliced or diced
(peaches, strawberries, apricots)
1 teaspoon maple syrup
Dash sea salt

Directions:
Simmer agar in juice and stir until dissolved.
Add syrup and salt.
Place fruit in a bowl or baking pan.
Pour mixture over fruit.
Refrigerate until firm (about three hours).
You can speed up the cooling if you place bowl with
mixture into a cold water bath for a few minutes
before refrigerating.

Tasha's Blueberry-Tahini Pudding

Kuzu, a starch made from the root of the kuzu plant, has
an alkalizing effect.

Ingredients:
2 cups blueberry juice
3 tablespoons kuzu
2 tablespoons tahini

Directions:
Dissolve kuzu in the blueberry juice.
Pour the mixture into a pan and cook on medium
heat for three minutes, stirring constantly.
Reduce heat to low and continue stirring until
thickened.
Remove from heat and fold in tahini.
Can be eaten cool or warm.

Change the amount of kuzu to alter the consistency.
Try pear or cherry juice for a different flavor.

Mark's Almond Milk

Ingredients:
    8 ounces organic raw almonds
    5 cups water

Directions:
    Place almonds in water and refrigerate for twelve to twenty-four hours.
    Rinse and combine in a blender with 5 cups of fresh water.
    Strain three times in a fine mesh stainless steel strainer, pushing through as much liquid as you can.
    Add enough water to make four cups.
    You could add a tablespoon or two of brown rice syrup or other sweetener if desired.

Other Snacks

Here are a few additional snacks you might want to try when the munchies hit.

Mochi – Found in the freezer section of your health food store these are cakes made from sweet brown rice. They're chewy and delicious when toasted and covered with your favorite spread. Cashew butter with a touch of jelly works well as the topping.
    Celery with almond butter
    Brown rice crackers with tahini
    Grain soother – Pour a little warm rice milk, or almond milk over a serving of your favorite grain, sprinkle with cinnamon, and add a touch of maple syrup or other sweetener.

Now that you've read through this section, you may want to decide on the healing protocol that makes the most sense and is most appealing to you, and stick to this protocol for seven days. If that feels too daunting, start with one day at a time. You may simply decide to make a few food-related adjustments, work with an imagery exercise, and treat yourself to a few minutes of Body Truth before going to bed. At the end of the day, review your choices and make the adjustments that feel most useful.

The most reliable test for judging whether you are truly engaged in the practices suggested in this book is this: If it begins to feel as though this is the most challenging, but also the most thrilling, mysterious, and rewarding assignment you've ever undertaken, chances are you're exactly where you need to be.

Busy Being Born

"…he not busy being born
is busy dying."

– Bob Dylan, *"It's Alright, Ma"*

Most women travel to Woodstock in a last-ditch effort to prop up their allegedly wilting ovaries, usually after years of unsuccessful medical treatment. Now they're three, five, even ten years older than when they first set out on this pilgrimage; they're worn out by disappointment, their endocrine systems rebelling against repeated prodding. Still, when I look through the names in my stack of sign-in books, and see how many women have gone on to conceive the old -fashioned way, I marvel at the resilience of the Holy Human Loaf.

The couples who do elect to use assisted reproduction credit their successes to the careful attention paid to internal cues and to an increased level of overall well-being.

The women who adopt view themselves as anything but "infertile." In fact, with so many of my students who choose this path, along with motherhood comes an unprecedented wave of creativity. It's as if the energy of childbirth gets channeled into ideas, projects, new beginnings.

Throughout our life we are continually presented with assignments. We may not have a choice in how and when they arrive, but we do have a choice in how we receive them. No matter how you ultimately resolve your desire for a child, my hope is that you remember to be unconditionally kind to yourself.

Your children are on their way: they're simply taking the scenic route, giving you a chance to remember that you too once arrived here on earth bearing a parcel filled with gifts. Your sons and daughters are making sure you get to unwrap and deliver a few more of those gifts before they show up.

Our fertility cannot be taken away from us. It is not based on our estradiol levels, or our ovarian reserve. It is based on our willingness to live a passionate, fruitful life, and to stay "busy being born."

Looking at My Daughter's Baby Picture

You smile
at my folly
that
once
I thought
It was
I
who needed to
give birth
to
you,
when all along
it was
you
who held me
tenderly
cupped
in your hand
descending
earthward
delivering
me
to life.

Acknowledgments

To the women and men who many years ago felt I had something of value to share, and to the others since then who have traveled to our Fertile Heart Studio, and who have written letters expressing appreciation and affection: There would be no book without you. My understanding of what it was that changed and saved my life became fully conscious through sharing it with you. I treasure the thought that books can bring strangers together as friends, because I love books myself and count as friends authors I have never met except through their work.

I feel a special debt of gratitude to the extraordinary women I've worked with who have given me permission to tell their story. May your courage and compassion bring countless blessings to you and to all those who will be strengthened by your stories..

Dr. Christiane Northrup's beautiful Foreword for *Inconceivable* and her continued support have been a huge gift. The fact that Dr. Northrup and her work are so respected and loved by so many people all over the world tells me that things are not as bleak as they sometimes appear to be.

To know Sparrow, is to love Sparrow. And to love his musings, and his brilliant and funny books, and late night e-mails that make me laugh out loud no matter how cranky I feel. I thank you, Sparrow, for being my teacher and good friend.

My perennial gratitude goes to the many teachers who have shown me the medicinal power of consistent kindness: Robert Wolf, Arnold Gallo, Moira and Bert Shaw, Ariel Goottblatt, Jason Shulman, Seth Fielding, Gerry Epstein, Carol Rose, Zoe Avstreih, Francis X. Clifton, Donny Maseng and many others who've shared their heart's wisdom with me over the years. (I first heard the story of Pythagoras from

Francis, and the story of the divine wisdom and the angels from Zoe.)

I most respectfully and gratefully acknowledge the many physicians, health care providers, authors and spiritual teachers who welcomed and validated my work: Elizabeth Lesser, Wayne Dyer, Bernie Siegel, Miriam Lieberman, Joseph Telushkin, Ellen Langer, Marc Goldstein, Carolyn Berger, Serafina Corsello, Niravi Payne, Jonathan Scher, Sami David, Richard Marrs, Mark Nesselson, Donielle Wilson, Rachel Koenig, Carol Hornig, Dylana Accola, Ken Frey, Melanie Murphy, Joyce Anastasi, Raymond Chang, Diane Allen, Cecille Barrington, Michael Snyter, Mitch Peritz, Yan Wu, Heidi Washburn, Rachel Bastow, Rita Bigel-Casher,Yosaif August.

Blessings on Oprah Winfrey, Lisa Sharkey, Stacey Strazis and Hazelle Goodman for their unceasing commitment to add to the Power of Kindness in the world, and for being instrumental in introducing my work to a larger audience.

The one thing every writer prays for is one reliably literate individual, who will offer the perfect ratio of judgment and appreciation. I couldn't have hoped for a more intelligent, and loving midwife to help coax this baby out than my dream of an editor, Sandy Dorr.

Many thanks to Tom Cherwin, and Cynthia Werthamer for their careful, and inspired copy editing, and for being such a pleasure to work with.

Mark Lerner's talent, patience, and good humor made picking a perfect dress for the Fertile Female into an adventure. Thank you for the beautiful jacket design, Mark.

I'm indebted to Janis Vallely for challenging me to shape eight years' worth of notes into the first draft of this book.

The resplendent community of Kehilat Lev Shalem, has become a most majestic soup kitchen for my starving soul.

Our beloved rabbi, Jonathan Kligler, has taught me that being Jewish is not only okay, but beautiful; that all spiritual traditions are essentially about filling the world with kindness.

Lillian and Miles Cahn, Judy and Gerry Miller, Lynn Francis, Rebecca Shippee, Bar Scott, Nick and Lillian Lenovits, Margie Jenkins, Sarah Zoogman, Jack Sharkey, Violet Snow, Viera and Marta Novak, Eli Noy, Juraj Gavora, Priscilla and James Lignori, Nancy and Jeff Langer, Rikki Asher, Royce Froelich, Janine Francolini, Nicky Silver, Linda Woznicki, Linda Harms, Dorothy Crystal Betsy Agoglia, John Beaulieu – friends and family who over the years have reached out to me during difficult times, gotten excited on my behalf, and delighted me by sharing their various adventures, their love of reading and writing, and their desire to keep searching. I most humbly thank each and every one of you for your generosity.

My sister Susan and brother-in-law Richard Diamond's open-armed hospitality toward all living creatures that cross their path, their love of learning, and their radical dedication to their children, and their elders, has amazed, and guided me over the last three decades.

Alexis, Matthew and Steven Diamond, my handsome, brilliant nephews, and three of the most decent human beings on.this planet, have cheered me on by forwarding relevant articles, offering feedback, building a swing in our backyard, loving their cousins, and mostly by gracing me with the gift of their presence in my life. They were the first to show me how loving a child can crack your heart wide open.

To the two beautiful beings Ellena and Adi, who landed here on earth to give Ed and me the delicious experience of parenting and who are an unending source of wonder: No Zen master could teach me more about being present

("If you're not going to be here, you might as well leave now, Mommy") and careful ("Watch it, Mom,the way you cut squash is the way you live your life!") the way you do. Being your mom is the sweetest of all my assignments.

To my husband, Edward Nathan Baum, I say here what he has heard me say time and again in the seventeen years of our marriage: You have taught me more about the meaning of pure heart, integrity, compassion, and permission, not to mention music, history, writing, cooking, and countless other arts, than I ever would have thought possible. Ours is surely an arranged marriage. In my mind's eye I see our mothers in the upper worlds beaming over the match they made.

One of my favorite teachings is based on a quote from Deuteronomy: "Choose life, so that you and your descendants may live." In other words, no matter what the circumstances, you must always choose the most life-enhancing attitude and course of action. My mother, Edita Lenorovich, and my father, Oskar Indich, continued to model for me throughout their event-filled lives what it means to keep "choosing life." If I ever accomplish anything worthwhile, the strength to have done so will have sprung from the deep well of their love.

I once heard a story of a spiritual teacher who worked with dying children. As the hour of their passing drew near, he would tell them to follow the light. "When the light goes left, you go left," he'd say. "Just follow the light." For my first thirty-eight years, shadows hovered over many of the events of my life. Yet somehow, in the midst of it all, the light kept breaking through, and I, too, was able to follow it. For that, Dear Light, I bow my head a thousand times a day and say, "Thank You!"

Selected Bibliography

Albom, Mitch. *The Five People You Meet in Heaven.* Hyperion, 2003.

Andrews, Lori B. *The Clone Age.* Henry Holt & Company, 2000.

Arem, Ridha. *The Thyroid Solution.* Ballantine Books, 1999.

Baroody, Theodore A. *Alkalize or Die.* Holographic Health Press, 1991.

Baum, Edward. *Unpublished manuscript of recipes and cooking suggestions.*

Berger, Gary, Marc Goldstein, and Mark Fuerst. *The Couple's Guide to Fertility.* Doubleday, 1995.

Berry, Wendell. *Life is a Miracle.* Counterpoint, 2000.

Bluestone, Sarvananda. *The World Dream Book.* Destiny Books, 2002.

Bly, Robert. *The Kabir Book.* Beacon Press, 1977.

Calbom, Cherie and Maureen Keane. *Juicing For Life.* Avery Publishing Group Inc., 1992.

Colbin, Annemarie. *Food and Healing.* Ballantine Books, 1996.

Colbin, Annemarie. *Food and Our Bones.* Plume, 1998.

Corsello, Serafina. The Ageless Woman. Corsello Communications, 1999.

Creech, Sharon. *Replay.* Harper Collins, 2005.

Daniels, Kaayla T. *The Whole Soy Story.* New Trends Publishing, Inc., 2005.

Diamond, Harvey, and Marilyn Diamond. *Fit for Life.* Warner Books, Inc., 1985.

Galland, Leo and Dian Dincin Buchman, *Superimmunity for Kids.* Copestone Press , Inc., 1988.

Gandhi, Mahatma. *Gandhi: An Autobiography.* Beacon Press 1993.

Goldberg, Burton. *Women's Health Series #1.* Future Medicine Publishing, 1998.

Grace, Matthew. *A Way Out.* Matthew Grace, 2000.

Heschel, Abraham Joshua. *God in Search of Man.* Farrar, Straus and Giroux, 1955.

Heschel, Abraham Joshua. *Moral Grandeur and Spiritual Audacity.* Farrar, Straus and Giroux, 1996.

Indichova, Julia. *Inconceivable.* Doubleday, 2001

Jung, C.G. *Memories, Dreams, Reflections.* Vintage Books, 1963.

Kierkegaard, Soren. *The Diary of Soren Kierkegaard.* Carol Publishing Group, 1993.

Lauersen, Neils H. and Colette Bouchez. *Getting Pregnant: What Couples Need to Know Right Now.* Fawcett Columbine, 1991.

Lesser, Elizabeth. *Broken Open:How Difficult Times Can Help Us Grow.* Villard, 2004.

Mann, John H. *Divine Androgyny.* Portal Press, 1999.

Marrs, Richard, Lisa Friedman Bloch, and Kathy Kirtland Silverman. *Dr. Richard Marrs' Fertility Book.* Dell, 1997.

Murray, Michael, Joseph Pizzorno, and Lara Pizzorno. *The Encyclopedia of Healing Foods.* Atria Books, 2005.

Northrup, Christiane. *Mother-Daughter Wisdom.* Bantam Books, 2005.

Nussbaum, Elaine. *Recovery from Cancer.* Avery Publishing Group Inc., 1992.

Oliver, Mary. *White Pine.* Harcourt, Inc., 1994.

Pert, Candace B. *Molecules of Emotion.* Touchstone, 1997.

Pitchford, Paul. *Healing with Whole Foods.* North Atlantic Books, 1993.

Pourafazal, Haleh, and Roger Montgomery. *The Spiritual Wisdom of Hafez.* Inner Traditions, 1998.

Rilke, Rainer Maria. *Letters to a Young Poet.* W. W. Norton

& Company, Inc., 1954.

Rudin, M.D., Donald and Clara Felix. *Omega-3 Oils*. Avery Publishing Group Inc. 1996.

Scher, M.D., Jonathon, and Carol Dix. *Preventing Miscarriage*. HarperCollins, 1991.

Shannon, Marilyn M. *Fertility, Cycles and Nutrition*. The Couple to Couple League International, Inc., 1996.

Tilberis, Liz. *No Time To Die*. Little, Brown & Company, 1998.

Walker, Dr. Norman W. *Colon Health*. Norwalk Press, 1979.

Watts, Alan. Out of the Trap. And Books, 1985.

Weed, Susan S. *Wise Woman Herbal for the Childbearing Year*. Ash Tree Publishing, 1986.

Weil M.D., Andrew. *Natural Health, Natural Medicine*. Houghton Mifflin Company, 1995.

Weschler, Toni. *Taking Charge of Your Fertility*. Harper Collins, 2001.

Wigmore, Ann. *The Wheatgrass Book*. Avery Publishing Group Inc., 1985.

Williamson, Marianne. *A Return to Love*. Harper Perennial, 1992.

The Tool Chest

Fertile Heart™ Imagery (CD)

Fertile Heart™ Imagery 2 (CD)

Fertile Heart™ Body Truth (CD)

Fertile Heart™ Chants Remedies (CD)

Exploring Holistic Fertility Treatment Options (CD)

For information about workshops, international phone-support circles, Guest Teacher Teleconferences with mainstream and integrative practitioners and more, please e-mail us at info@fertileheart.com.

Julia Indichova and the Fertile Heart™ community hope to raise awareness about the work of the organizations listed below, and many other national organizations doing similar work.

Turn It Around Project www.turnitaroundproject.org
The Beehive Collective www.beehivecollective.org
Physicians for Social Responsibility www.psr.org
Heifer International www.heifer.org
Habitat for Humanity www.habitat.org
Environmental Defense www.environmentaldefense.org

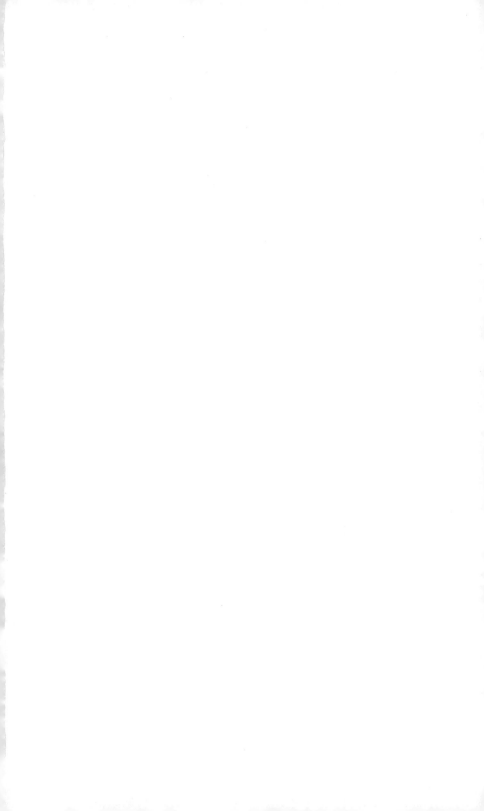